"THE UNSUNG HEROES OF TRA[...]
en who created safe spaces for us to e[...]
championed our rights. Thanks to true feminist allies like Veronica Vera, fledgeling trans women and other people needing to break out of the straitjacket of masculinity have had a safe place to discover a more liberated self." – Zackary Drucker, artist, co-producer of *Transparent*

"VERONICA IS ONE OF MY FAVORITE SEX AUTHORS. She taught me that gender is like a sex role – like being on stage in costume. My current role is being an outrageous granny publicly supporting and teaching masturbation all the way to the bank. Warning: Once I started reading I couldn't stop!" – Betty Dodson, www.dodsonandross.com, pioneering sex educator

"A REAL WORK OF HEART, welcoming loving partners into the often painfully private art of cross dressing. This relationship-positive book will teach you how to make cross-dressing a shared sexy, intimate, guilt and shame-free adventure that promises growth and transformation for everyone involved. Brava, Miss Vera!" – Barbara Carrellas, author, *Ecstasy is Necessary*

"VERONICA VERA'S WORK WITH GENDER IS UNIQUE and full of compassion about human possibility. Regardless of your own identity, you can explore the insights and delights of gender play with her engaging new guidebook. – Carol Queen, PhD, co-founder & director, Center for Sex & Culture, and co-author of *The Sex & Pleasure Book*

"THIS BOOK IS A JOYFUL CELEBRATION of gender expression and love. Veronica Vera's shares her decades of experience and her personal brand of 'Frock Therapy' to liberate the cross-gender spirit in us all." – Kit Rachlin, Ph.D. psychologist & gender specialist

Miss Vera's Cross Gender Fun For All

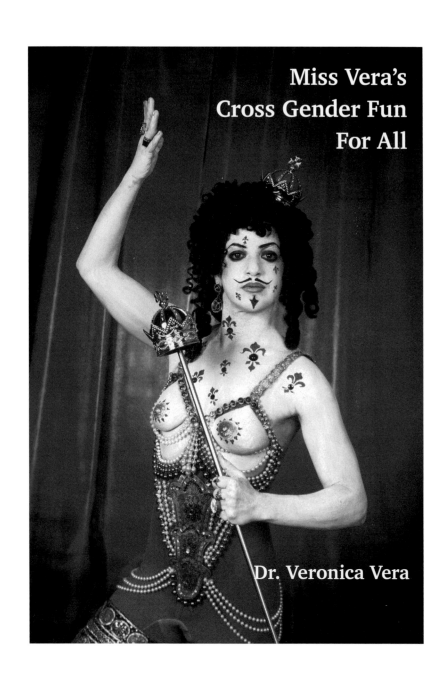

Miss Vera's
Cross Gender Fun
For All

Dr. Veronica Vera

Cover by Johnny Ink, www.johnnyink.com.

Cover photograph by Hana Pesut.

Illustrations by Kate Devereux Smith.

Title page photograph of Shelly Mars, Queen of Clubs, by Annie Sprinkle.

Published in the United States by Greenery Press. Distributed by SCB Distributors, Gardena, CA.

THIS BOOK IS DEDICATED TO ARTISTS OF LIFE,

ESPECIALLY

STUART "MISTY MADISON" COTTINGHAM

AND CANDICE "CANDIDA ROYALLE" VADALA

CONTENTS

CONTENTS

INTRODUCTION

ARE YOU A MAN who's been in a situation and thought, "If only I were a woman, things would be so different"? Or, if you're a woman, have you thought, "This would not have happened if I were a man"? Who would you be, if even for a day, you could be your gender opposite, and go from male to female or female to male? Which aspects of your life do you feel would benefit if you could reach within yourself to find this "other," learn from the experience and use it?

Look around. On the street, on television and the Internet, in schools and colleges... perhaps you yourself, or someone within your family... individuals, with the aid of science, chemistry, fashion and community, transcend gender lines to literally change the face and figure of society. After years of pioneers' efforts, transgender culture has gone from underground to mainstream, its visibility aided by high profile trans people with access to the media.

Cher cheered and millions of television viewers watched her son Chaz Bono, once known as her daughter Chastity, compete on *Dancing With The Stars*. Trans woman Laverne Cox, a star of the hit series *Orange Is The New Black,* became an eloquent spokesperson for the trans community and graced the cover of *Time Magazine*. These and others are significant revelations, but none more startling than the debut of Caitlyn Jenner – as the former Bruce Jenner, Olympic decathlon winner, once called the world's strongest man – became the world's most fascinating woman.

If you don't identify as transgender, you might think our world has gone mad. Perhaps you struggle to understand. To me, this shift makes absolute sense: within every man there is a woman; within every woman there is a man. As the founder of Miss Vera's Finishing School for Boys Who Want to Be Girls, the world's first transgender academy, I prove this with men and women every day.

This book is a practical guide to cross gender transformation – whether your intentions are serious, playful or both. As long as you are curious, there is information for you.

My goal in the main section of this book is to inform you, as well as to stimulate your thinking. The resource section, at the end, provides starting points to begin your own investigations. Besides the individual items, there may be categories you never even considered. Let the adventure begin!

PART ONE

BYE-BYE BINARY

L ET'S THINK ABOUT THE DAYS of the caves, when gender roles were determined simply by our need for survival. Sex and gender were considered one and the same. The male of the species was built bigger and stronger. He hunted for food, and he planted his seed to ensure the growth of the tribe. The female of the species carried the seed and nurtured the young. Each was a protector in their own way. There wasn't much time for anything else. Individuals mated, mates formed families, families formed tribes. Society was born and things speeded up fast. As society advanced, everything expanded: our bodies, including our brains, got bigger; as did our opportunities for work, for leisure, for learning, for connections to each other, for happiness and for stress, the main stress being fear of death.

We created religions that could not save us from death, but promised a happy afterlife, if we only we followed the rules – which were based on the gender binary. We've hung on to that tired old binary because we connect it to our survival. Our adherence to gender-binary thinking has continued long after the need for those restricted divisions has disappeared. Meanwhile, the fabric of society is bursting at the seams.

We are all aware that the lines between genders have blurred: women have moved from the bedroom to the boardroom; men have proved themselves to be highly capable homemakers and childcare providers. This is about more than who wears the pants and who dons the apron.

Clothing is not simply about fabric. Clothing has always been connected to the way in which we experience and identify gender. The act of cross-dressing, wearing clothing of the opposite sex, changes what we project as well as what we interpret about others. Never just a fashion statement, nor only about pleasure, cross-dressing is about liberation, expansion, and a shift in power.

The awareness of cross gender options which cross-dressing facilitates is not for trans folk alone. Cross-dressing is part of a much bigger picture; it is something from which we can all benefit, even more than you may already have.

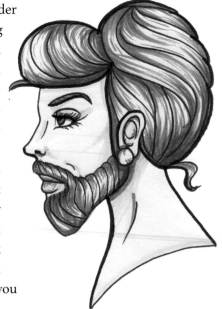

I have provided you with questions and explanations that help you to go deeper than your clothes, or your make-up, or even your body. I dare you to peel back the layers and reveal parts of you that lie dormant. No matter who you are or how you identify, I invite you to develop your own cross gender identity, and then create a symbol to remind you. That symbol can be a tiny item you carry with you or keep nearby, or you can follow the instructions, using props, clothing and make-up for a full body cross gender transformation. That item or photo of that cross gender identity will then be an icon, a constant reminder of the fullness of your humanity.

Cross Gender Fun for All

I **AM PRIVILEGED** to be in a very unique position as the dean of Miss Vera's Finishing School for Boys Who Want to Be Girls. For more than twenty years, I and my faculty of deans, all experts in aspects of femininity, have helped those who live in the male role explore the women they feel inside. In my academy studio we use clothing and make-up to perform a physical transformation.

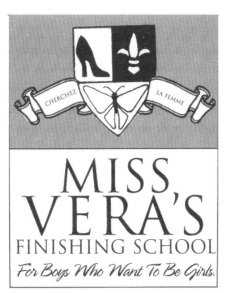

But we don't stop there. I devise a program that involves practical lessons and field trips to expand each student's world. In the process, by transforming the body, I enter the world of the mind. I have made discoveries that

Miss Vera's Finishing School crest.
Design by Viqui Maggio

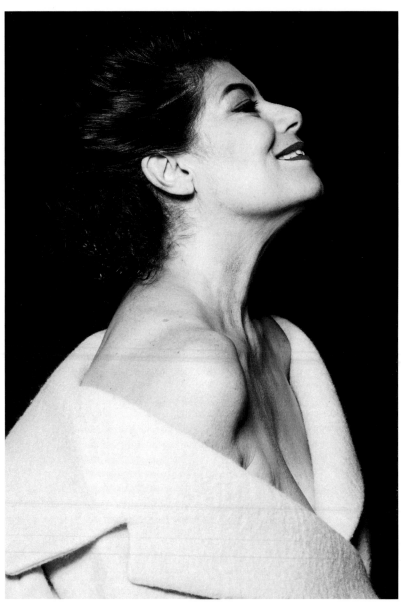

Miss Vera, dean of students. Photo by Philippe Vogelenzang.

Cross Gender Fun for All

psychologists have told us about for years. In interviews, I've referred to what we do as therapy with props (I've jokingly used the term "Frock Therapy").

The results of my academy's efforts are exciting, but no joke, and they have very positive effects. I've helped some students strengthen their relationships and helped others find new ones. We've uncovered hidden talents, relieved sexual inhibitions, inspired better levels of health. Our students begin to understand and accept those parts of their selves that were hidden, and developed others more fully. There have been a few times when our efforts produced unpleasant results, when the student was simply not ready to grow in self-acceptance – but those experiences, though not always pleasant, were just as informative. Our goal is the same as that of traditional therapy: we strive for a fully integrated human being who has more options. But Miss Vera's frock therapy is more fun. And you can do it, too.

Cross Gender Fun for All

WHAT'S SEX GOT TO DO WITH IT?

WHAT'S SEX GOT TO DO WITH IT?

WHEN I BEGAN MY SCHOOL, many of the people who enrolled had never shared their desire to cross dress and find the woman inside with anyone. The constraints of the gender binary defined sex and gender as the same thing and heterosexuality as the norm. This kind of thinking labeled anyone outside those so-called norms as immoral. Because sexual pleasure, especially masturbation, has often been a way to access these hidden parts of themselves, these visitors to my academy had learned to conceal feelings that a sex-negative society had labeled weird and perverse.

I am sex-positive. For me, your sexual practice is not a road to ruin, but yet another path to enlightenment. The way you understand your sexual needs, desires, and actions is an essential guide to self-acceptance and empowerment.

Fortunately, society has become more educated and understanding. Not only gender benders, but all kinds of minorities have found more inclusion and support. In 2015, the U.S. Supreme Court allowed for same-sex marriage; trans people are free to serve in the military; Amnesty International took a stand in favor of the decriminalization of prostitution. We live in a time of great healing, and this is reflected in the progress made by trans gender people. In exploring your options, we'll talk about gender, but we'll also talk about sexuality, because that is an essential part of this discussion and to the Miss Vera method.

I'd grown up in a loving family, but one ruled by religious precepts that I could not follow and still feel true to myself. I was told masturbation was bad, because "God does not like that," and girls who had sex before marriage were whores. It was either accept these religious rules on blind faith and stay a (frustrated) virgin until marriage, break the rules and be condemned to hell... or trust my natural inclinations, follow my desires, live out my fantasies and find my own answers.

Manhattan called to me like the Emerald City. In August, 1970, five thousand women marched down Fifth Avenue in the First Women's March for Equality. Less than a year before, I had arrived in New York to get a job in publishing. But I couldn't type. Gender roles were tight, and as a woman, every entry level job required typing, so I wound up in Wall Street as a stock trader's assistant. There, I didn't need to type, just be pretty and charming over the phone during office hours and after work at cocktail time.

Despite the Women's March, sexual harassment ran rampant. Like many young women, I could not recognize when it was happening, or that it was happening to me.

By the end of the '70s, a lot had changed for women. Our consciousness was raised; we had access to the birth control pill. The '60s cultural revolution was a wave that entered the '70s and by the end of that decade brought liberation to many minorities: blacks, women, and sexual minorities. By that time, I had happily relieved myself of my virginity many times over.

MY SEXUAL EVOLUTION

MY SEXUAL EVOLUTION

WHEN MY MOM DIED in 1979, it was a wake-up call. I decided to leave the world of high finance and pursue my dream to be a writer. The only person I knew who was working in the field was at Penthouse Publications, editing a journal called *Variations* that contained stories of a mind-boggling list of sexual activities: swinging, cunnilingus, fellatio, frotteurism, bondage.

Through that first writing gig, I met others who believed in sexual information over sexual ignorance. Human sexuality became my field of study.

I tried everything, did everything and wrote about it. I made a few hardcore adult movies and kinky videotapes, collaborated with other artists such as Robert Mapplethorpe and Annie Sprinkle, advocated for the decriminalization of prostitution, testified for freedom of expression before a committee of the U.S Senate in Washington, D.C. I evolved as a human being because I embraced that deepest, supposedly darkest part of myself, my sexuality. I found friends and mentors and colleagues with whom I could be my true self. Because of this, my spirit prospered.

With all of this experience, I decided to write a memoir of those years and my sexual evolution. My academy, "Miss Vera's Finishing School for Boys Who Want to Be Girls," began as a way to help finance the writing of that memoir. I came up with a big idea – a school where men could learn to be women – at a time when gender roles were in an extreme state of flux. My experiences and research had given me confidence and clarity so that in the early '90s, when the media asked me to explain the transgender issues of our student body, I was ready.

Those who present themselves at my academy are on a journey of self-discovery and personal liberation, just as I had been. News of Miss Vera's Finishing School took off and my academy has become known throughout the world. A few thousand students have studied on campus, and many thousands more have read my two previous books. I am grateful for all of their testimonials.

Our efforts have caused a ripple effect. A good portion of our students inspired by their experience have become activists themselves – through commitments of time, money or both.

What I have experienced through my students has taught me a lot. I choose not to censor dreams, but to facilitate them. This process of cross gender exploration, which has proven so helpful to so many, is a boon to all.

Male and female are defined as gender opposites, dependent on each other for survival. There is a third gender and it is trans, but it could not exist without male and female. Trans people are change personified. It's not only transgender people who benefit in this age of gender fluidity. I believe these discoveries are of benefit to all. I'm excited to share them with you.

Call it madness, if you like, but there is a method to this madness, the Miss Vera Method of Self Discovery and Growth through Cross Gender Play.

WHY THIS BOOK
AT THIS TIME?

T O RING IN the age of gender fluidity.

To foster love and unity among people.

To disarm the battle of the sexes.

To demonstrate the connection between sexuality and gender.

To inspire you with our Academy success stories.

To strengthen your relationships – those that exist, and those yet to be formed.

To share with you what I learned through my marriage to a transgender person.

To embrace my status as a doctor of human sexuality and acknowledge my expanded understanding of the benefits of that work.

To develop my own cross gender identity and icon.

To appreciate the transgender phenomenon as art in life.

To examine the role of fashion in culture.

To provide you with instructions on the physical transformations.

To have fun.

Cross Gender Fun for All

HE PLAYED MISTY FOR ME

HE PLAYED MISTY FOR ME

AMONG THE LIST OF REASONS to write this book at this time, the most personal is because I married Stuart Ira Cottingham.

　　We met at the *bon voyage* party of our mutual friend, Stephanie. Stu had dated her; she was my good friend and neighbor. At the time, I was preparing to launch another session of

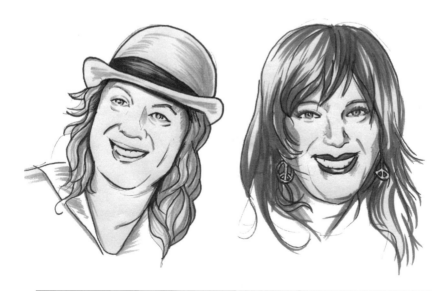

our academy group lesson in "How to Walk In High Heels," a class for all who identify as women: cross-dressers, trans women and cis women (the term popularized by author and transgender activist Julia Serrano to denote non-trans women). I knew quite a few of Stephanie's girl friends, and they were aware of my academy, so I told them about the upcoming lesson.

"Are you going to have those guys in dresses in class with us women?" asked one of the cis guests.

"Well, it's not really accurate to call them 'guys in dresses'," I explained, "because when they are dressed, they feel very deeply that they *are* women."

It was the first time that I had put it so strongly. When I first began my academy, I was careful not to refer to the men who arrived at our door as women. They had not had the same life experience as genetic women; I did not want to offend cis women. But at this point, I was fifteen years into my work with academy students and I had a much greater understanding of the people who came to me.

I was very pleased when a voice behind me called out, "Right on." The good-looking fellow who had spoken came up, thrust out his hand and introduced himself: "Hi, I'm Stu Cottingham."

"It's very interesting that you supported what I said," I told him, "because I've never put it so strongly before."

"Well," said Stu, "I'm bisexual and I cross dress sometimes."

After dealing with so many closet cases for so many years, Stu's words were a breath of fresh air. I've helped many students find the woman inside, but not everyone shares that knowledge with the people closest to them.

Stu identified his femmeself as "Misty." He said that Misty was part of his sexual nature. Both Stu and Misty became my friends and then my lovers.

On our very first date, I had asked Stu a question that seemed to come out of nowhere, unless you consider the people involved: "What do you think about your penis?" You see, in my experience as dean of the world's first transgender academy, I've learned that if you tell me you are not happy with your penis and would prefer it not be there, there is a good chance you may one day transition.

I've had sex with transwomen and transmen, with cis women, and with cis men… but my coupled relationships have been with men comfortable to be penis owners, and I did not expect that to change in the near future. I just wanted to know what I was getting into.

"Well, I'm Jewish," Stu said, "so I wish my penis were a little bigger, but I like it. I don't want to get rid of my penis." Question answered.

I had yet to meet Misty, and the time when I would meet her was growing closer. My experience, as well as the answers students gave on their enrollment applications, told me that the majority of the men who come to my Academy would love to have their femininity accepted by their partners during lovemaking. „I know when I meet Misty, we are going to have sex," I told Stu.

"Oh, first time with Misty… that will be interesting." Stu was intrigued and Misty was excited. Both were nervous. I decided that I

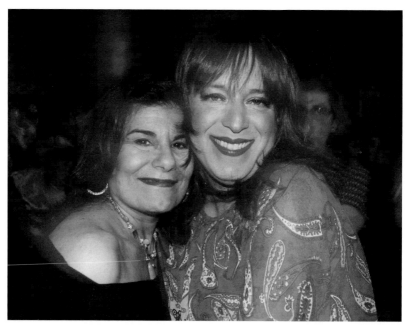

Veronica and Misty Madison. Photo by Cory Mervis.

would go to Stu's apartment and he would have Misty ready to greet me, which meant he would put her together himself. What would I, the doyenne of cross dressing, think of Misty?

She opened the door and we both let out a sigh of relief. Misty could read the approval in my eyes. She looked really cute. Stu was an artist. His talent served him well in the choice of Misty's red wig and the way he did her make-up. She wore a very short denim skirt, red fishnets and a red nylon off-the-shoulder halter, *à la* Daisy Duke. We listened to music and Misty danced for me. Then we danced together... from the living room to the bedroom.

That first time, we made love for five hours. We took a dinner break in the middle. Went out for something light, a couple slices of pizza, then back.

When we returned from outdoors, Stu was no longer dressed in Misty mode, but Misty was still in his head and the heat that had been generated returned as soon as we lay down and touched, skin to skin. Misty's large clitoris, or "girl cock," was put to use. I would learn that Stu was a versatile lover but Misty's preference for giving pleasure was through oral sex, and she excelled.

Many of my students who have female partners have confided they love to give their wives and girlfriends oral pleasure. Misty's big luscious red lips lapped me up and drank me in as I came and she came and he came. Oh, it was grand.

We didn't become a couple right away. There were a few obstacles. Stu was eighteen years my junior and still hoped to have children. I was beyond child-bearing. I looked forward to a partner with lots of stability, i.e. a rich guy; Stu was a hippie at heart. But we let our love and our trust develop. Soon those other things just did not matter as much as what we had.

Since I make a practice to not date my students, Misty was never officially enrolled, but she audited plenty. She learned a lot, but the most important lesson in life Stu learned before he ever met me, and that was self-acceptance. He recounted a story about his dad Robert, and his Aunt JoAnn. One day JoAnn came to her big brother and confided that she was attracted to women. Bob suggested they take out the dictionary and look up the word "love." "You see, it doesn't say anything here about love needing to being only about a man and a woman," said Stu's dad. Stu was so proud that his father, a kid living in rural Indiana in 1924, could have such an open-minded attitude. Stu adored and admired his dad, and even more important, he emulated his dad's tolerance and understanding. These are traits so worth teaching to younger generations. I emphasize this when students tell me they fear discovery by their own children. Do they want to perpetuate the same world they grew up in? Stu's self-confidence and acceptance of Misty, his cross gender alter ego, was amazingly attractive. We were compatible in every way we held dear.

We made love and we shared fantasies. Stu shared his with me more easily than I shared mine with him. I could say that as a porn star, I'd lived out many of my fantasies, but that wasn't accurate. I'd had many lovers and many wild sexual experiences, the memories of which still fueled some of my fantasies. But I was less inclined to let him or any lover know the parade of images that passed through my brain as I drew close to orgasm. I think women are more reluctant to share that information.

But Misty loved to imagine herself the prize awarded to winners of a battle, usually a battle between mismatched opponents where the smaller of the two men was getting the worst of it, until he suddenly turned the tide and knocked the stuffing out of the big guy. Misty still liked being the big guy's girlfriend, even if he lost.

She fantasized that I was her queen and she one of my sexy handmaidens. I sat on an imaginary throne and spread my legs, giving my handmaidens instructions to pleasure me. I came to love that role, the woman in charge, the Sapphic queen. This was a new persona for me.

In my own wet dreams I was the one taken, ravaged, more passive. Misty loved to be taken, but she was a more lusty wench, she'd put up a fight, a man had to win this treasure.

Stu's bisexuality meant that Misty enjoyed sex with men, but Stu's relationship partners, both sexual and emotional, were women. To Misty, men were instruments of pleasure, not meant for commitment.

I understood the difference between sex in a committed relationship and sex for fun. I had learned so much from exploring my own sexual issues, I did not feel threatened when Stu explored his. In fact, I felt that was part of what made us so compatible.

Misty continued to be part of our lovemaking, but in a more subtle way. There was often a moment when Stu and I made love when I heard a slight change in the sound of his breathing and I knew though we were both naked, Misty was with me. So, like Scheherazade, I described a captivating scene, and won my love's heart.

After five extraordinary years together, we set our wedding date for June, 9, 2012. We began to practice our first dance as a married couple, and we chose "Misty" as our song; after all it was Misty who brought us together. But, alas, our dance was not to be a long one. Just one month before our wedding Stu was diagnosed with a deadly brain tumor. We had only ten more months. They were challenging months, but months filled with joy and love. Stu treated every day of those ten months as a gift. He received and radiated love. Our time was joyful until the very last. My husband left the planet an even more enlightened being, and I felt blessed to have shared such great love.

If we were not meant to grow old together, why had fate brought us to each other? What was the message here? How would I take the power of that love and keep it alive? What had I learned that I could impart to others?

What if Stu had lived and continued to be Misty? What if he had transitioned? I had asked myself that question a few times. Was it so far-fetched? Not long after we became lovers, Stu had confided he was considering surgery – not sexual reassignment surgery, but a butt lift. He'd actually gone to a plastic surgery, gotten an estimate, and was about to sign on the dotted line so that he, and Misty, could have prominent buttocks. The recovery process would have taken many weeks in a body cast, not a helpful prospect for our budding romance.

I suggested a padded panty. Fortunately for us both, he took my advice, and that gave our love time to grow.

By the time we were deeply in love, I knew it wouldn't have mattered if he had transitioned. I loved Stu and I loved Misty. But what about early on, when I asked myself that same question? Although I had enjoyed sex with women, I didn't like the idea that my primary relationship would be with a female partner. When I examined why, I realized it was because I wanted to be the "girl," not be in competition with her. I wanted to be the pretty one, the one who got the man; the one who was protected; the one who got the flowers. I was stuck in the muck of the gender binary.

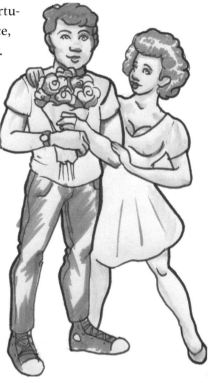

If Stu had not been so honest with me right from the start... if I had not been so sexually experienced and knowledgeable, so respectful and accepting of his differences... had we not found ways that could work for us both... our love might have been buried. Instead, we did not fall in love, we rose in love, and love lifted us higher. This journey of sexual self-discovery is one important part of what I want to share with you. Cross gender play is the delightful path we will take.

CALLING
DR. VERA

S HORTLY AFTER APRIL 20, 2013, the one-year anniversary of my husband's passing, I learned I was to be awarded the degree Doctor of Human Sexuality from the Institute for the Advanced Study of Human Sexuality in San Francisco. Founded in 1968, an outgrowth of the Sexual Revolution, IASHS was the first school to award advanced degrees in sexuality, thus recognizing sexuality as a branch of knowledge worthy of its own discipline and creating the professional field of sexology. The first dean of the school was Wardell Pomeroy, a member of Alfred Kinsey's research team. The current dean and a founder is Dr. Ted McIlvenna, a true visionary.

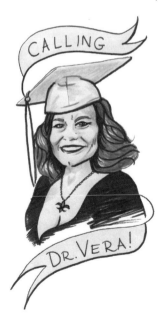

In June, I travelled to San Francisco to be invested with my degree. It was an especially joyous occasion because it was also a reunion with my best friends, the women of Club 90, Jane Hamilton, Candida Royalle and Annie Sprinkle, the first porn star support group which we formed with Gloria Leonard in 1983. In recognition of our life's work, Dr. McIlvenna would award not only me, but Jane and Candida with doctoral degrees; Gloria would receive hers posthumously. Annie had achieved her Ph.D. from the IASHS in 2002.

During our investiture ceremony, Dr. Ted remarked, "During every revolution, there are those who have a revelation." He referred to us as having had revelations. Candida had pioneered the field of erotica by and for women and couples; Jane was a "love missionary" to China, teaching the women there sexual self-esteem; Gloria had championed free speech and feminism; Annie was a performance artist who with her partner Beth Stephens founded "Ecosex," in which the earth was not mother, but lover.

Have you ever heard someone speak words that you felt in your heart but had never dared speak? Dr. Ted's words really resonated with me. My work in sexuality and gender has always been so far from what I ever expected I would do, it has felt like a revelation, a calling.

That doctorate could not have come at a better time. This was the perfect catalyst to help me move forward with my life and my work, following the death of my husband.

I used the home page of our academy website to invite couples to visit, so that I could help other couples understand each other the way Stu and I did. "Build it and they will come." Now that the female partners are more involved, I see that cross gender play is helpful to both partners, individually and in the context of their relationship. Just as a person living in the male role is happy when we help reveal the woman within, so his female partner can benefit from exploring her inner man.

When I founded my academy, I did so with the idea that I wanted to put more female energy into the world, that there needed to be a shift in power from male domination. I still do believe that, but now I see that on an individual basis, each of us has our own need for balance.

Sometimes a student will tell me that he is a husband who loves to buy clothes for his wife. "I shop for all her clothes," he'll boast. However, that student will often express frustration because while his own femme persona loves the full skirts and high heels he adds to his wife's wardrobe, the wife's response is far from enthusiastic. It occurred to me that the wife simply might not share her husband's taste.

After meeting more and more spouses I realized while some of the wives preferred ultra-femme styles, others might like to butch it up. So I offer couples a complete role reversal: he to she and she to he.

Sometimes you and a partner may have somehow lost the spark that you once had. Cross gender play can be a fun way to improve communications, to reconnect and re-ignite that flame.

My academy process has worked well with those who want to access the qualities they identify as female, and now helps women who want to access more qualities they identify as male. What about me? How do I envision my male alter ego? What can I learn and how can I benefit from my own Mr. Right?

You say you have no burning desire, but are curious to see how you might benefit from gender play: then I invite you to discover your cross gender self.

Cross Gender Fun for All

JUNG AT HEART TЯAƎH TA ƏИUႱ

MY DOCTORATE WAS MORE than a certificate, it was more than the recognition of others; it expanded my thinking about how intricately our sexual practice is woven into our lives. It also brought me back to the thoughts I had when I first began the work of Miss Vera's Finishing School.

The school had begun as a sideline. As a favor to a friend, I had helped a few cross-dressers with their hair and make-up. One in particular, a 38-year-old attorney who went by "Sally Sissyribbons," was under my tutelage for an entire weekend.

Encouraged by my success with Sally and others, and needing to find a way to supplement my income while I worked on a memoir about my personal sexual evolution, I placed an ad in a tabloid called *Transvestian*. Once the phone began to ring, I learned the callers all wanted the same things: to find the women they felt themselves to be, inside.

What these men want is not impossible, I thought. *They need a school, a finishing school. But not for girls. A finishing school for boys who want to be girls.*

The name was a stroke of genius for which I am grateful. It was fun and funny, and right to the point. It was shameless.

The name was also the concept. I would create a school with lessons and a faculty where people could learn and grow. The men who came to me were looking for their "anima," the woman inside.

Psychologist Carl Jung had coined the term "collective unconscious" to describe the mental structures shared by all humans. Each man has a feminine unconscious mind, his *anima*. Each woman has a male unconscious mind, her *animus*. You can think of these as buried memories.

I had set up Miss Vera's Finishing School in ways that made sense in order for my students to accomplish goals and grow from the experience. Little did I realize that every way in which I chose to organize my academy program followed the basic steps of Jungian analysis: confession – which I prefer to call acknowledgement – elucidation, education and transformation. The curriculum designed for academy students would be relevant for everybody.

The name of the school is fun, accessible, right to the point. Anyone opting to make contact acknowledged their desire to go from male to female.

Back then, I understood that the students who came to me were merely the tip of an iceberg. They reflected a need that I called Venus Envy. Some wanted to live as women for a day, others for a lifetime, and many others were undecided.

Was I encouraging a band of male defectors? No, I was giving people more options.

When women felt the need to share more in the male experience, we created the women's movement. I thought this put women ahead of the game in terms of personal opportunities.

But life is a dynamic process. Yes, opportunities for women are greater than ever but whether male or female, this need for balance between who we are as humans, who we aspire to be, what messages have been imparted to us, and what we need to learn in order to grow, requires constant vigilance. We are not always prepared to seize or even recognize our opportunities – sometimes it helps to step outside ourselves and be someone new. So let's get started.

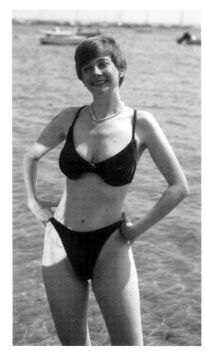 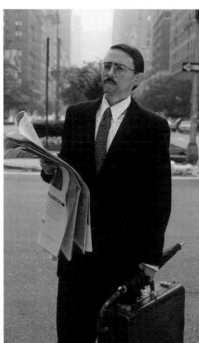

Katharine Gates and Katharine as Edwin Rochester III. Photos by Annie Sprinkle.

YOU AND YOUR ICON

THE PROCESS OF CREATING your cross gender identity and symbol requires your imagination. If you can dream it, you can be it.

This iconic *other* will serve as your guardian angel, your personal champion, your inner slut - whatever you need to feel balance in your life. Through the tried and true Miss Vera Method,

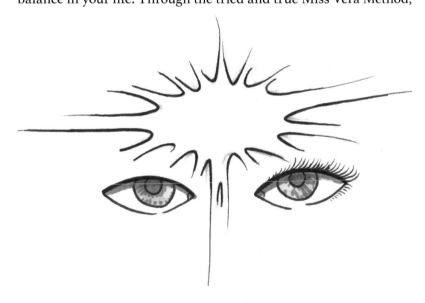

we will use clothing, props, instructions, exercises, and photos to bring your "other" to light.

The mirror might not reflect what you see in your imagination; mirrors rarely do. But I want you to look with your third eye, your mind's eye. You can follow the step by step process that I outline here, or make small changes.

Sometimes a tiny change can make a gigantic difference: polish one finger or go for a complete mani-pedi. Change that pretty wallet to a dark leather billfold. Where we go from there depends on what you hope to accomplish.

The first step for any prospective student of Miss Vera's Finishing School is completion of the enrollment application, so I've devised one just for you. This enrollment application helps you to define your goals – whether they involve work or play, or are task- or pleasure-oriented – and to recognize the steps you need to accomplish those goals. A graduation picture is a must. Photograph your cross gender identity or that symbol. The photo is for you as further inspiration, but extra credit goes to those who send me a copy.

THE TRANSFORMATION from male to female is not an end in itself, though that first look in the mirror is a pivotal moment; it is simply the first step in self-acceptance. We have put clothes on the student's psyche, made visible what before was only a feeling. We have made a dream come true.

For some students, this is as far as they will go; they are not ready to share this part of themselves with others. That is why I say this next step in the transformation and your

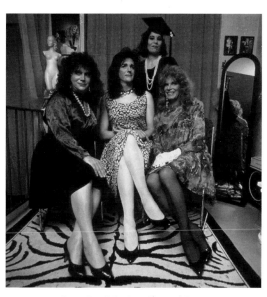

Joan, Patricia, Jennifer and Dean Vera. Photo by Abe Frajndlich.

cross gender play is the most challenging. In order to grow, it's important to let this new self blossom. If it's a sexual feeling, find it a partner or partners. If it's a talent, put it to use. If it's an emotion, release it. In that way, you become more of your self.

In the case of many of our students we succeeded, and with that success came the students' realizations that they were not simply masculine or feminine, that they could not fully realize themselves as human unless they stepped outside the gender binary, because that concept no longer fit. It also helped to step out of the house.

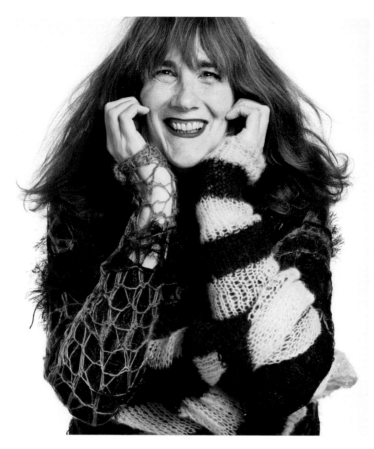

Patricia Harrington. Photo by Philippe Vogelenzang.

Patricia – who enrolled as Pat, a gloomy pessimist – blossomed into a transgender activist ready to help change the world. Patricia is on staff at Transgender Legal Defense.

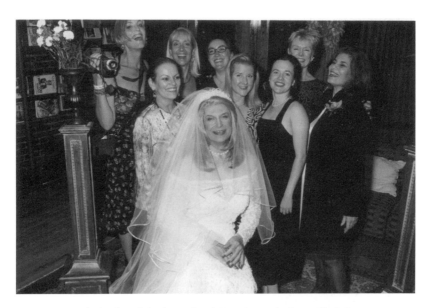

Bride Gayle and the deans (l to r) Kate Bornstein, Irene Clark, Bar-bara Carrellas, Eva Pendleton, Deborah Raposa, Melissa Hope, Maryann Byington, Miss Vera. Photo by wedding guest.

Prior to his first visit, John lived in the closet alone in his wedding gown. He loved his wife, but did not share with her for fear he would cause her pain. We transformed him to Gayle and created Gayle's wedding, complete with a groom, festive reception and a wedding video. It took a few years before John screwed up the courage to share Gayle's beautiful wedding video with his wife. His wife accepted her husband's need for Gayle and, moreover, she accepted Gayle's need for a boyfriend. They all became friends. The last time John and his wife came to New York, I had dinner with John, his wife and Gayle's boyfriend.

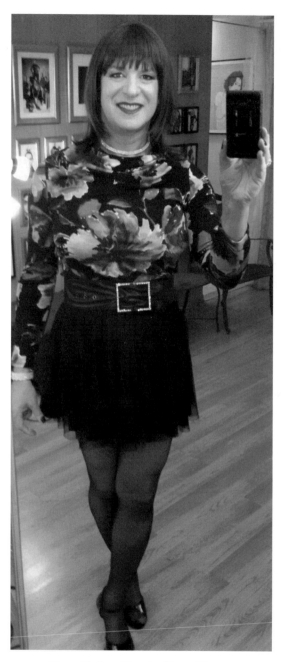

Ginger Liscious. Photo by Ginger Liscious.

Ned's successful career in sales netted him an early retirement. He then spent a few years in isolation, spending long days as Ginger. Ginger wrote to me in 2011, but it wasn't until 2014 that we actually met.

Ned was ready and eager to study on a fast track. Within eighteen months Ginger came out in a national magazine; Ned dealt with childhood traumas and re-united with family members. Ned shared Ginger with those closest to him; his criterion for new friends are those from whom he doesn't have to hide Ginger. Ned likes living in both worlds. He's coming out of retirement to embark on a brand new career as a motivational speaker.

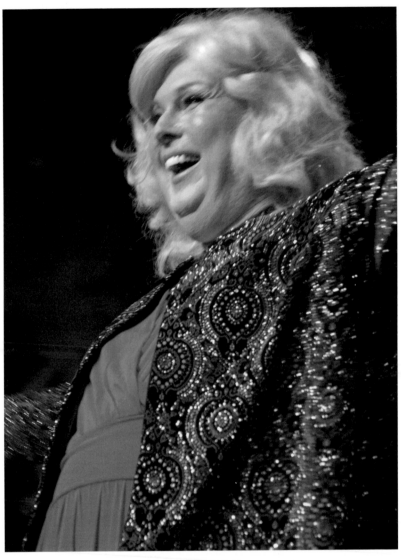
A very happy Chrissy Sue. Photo by Cory Mervis.

When Jim who was Chrissy Sue shared her trans identity with the sister whom she had not seen for twenty years, she learned her sister had run away from home because she was a lesbian. The siblings reunited and formed a new family. In 2010 Chrissy Sue published her autobiography, *Come Out, Come Out, Whoever You Are.*

- Stu as a young boy had sung in the children's choir of NY Metropolitan Opera until his voice changed. Misty began taking singing lessons in preparation for a solo show as a hippie chick.

- Chris reported that he never again felt intimidated at a corporate meeting since Christina had been to high tea in high drag at the Plaza hotel.

- Numerous students have become more diet conscious in order to feel more attractive in their feminine clothes.

- Ken wanted desperately to serve his wife as her maid, Ruth. I encouraged Ken's wife to find a new female persona for herself. She decided to be Elizabeth, a woman who was European-born and accustomed to being served by others. The couple learned to role-play and rekindled their romance.

Because of other personal considerations – young children, job security – it has taken years before a student will fill the dreams they have brought to my academy. We are an important stepping stone. Privacy is still an important consideration for many of my students. Though I know most of their legal names, I respect that privacy. Student Jennifer Summers was so grateful for her experience she gave permission for me to publish her photo in my second book, *Miss Vera's Cross Dress For Success*. She left the academy and remained very supportive of our efforts. In 2013, when billionaire Jennifer Natalya Pritzker announced her transition, I was happy for my student Jennifer Summer, a former paratrooper. I was proud of the dignified way the announcement was accomplished, despite her high profile. "We're not surprised" was the simple quote given by those closest to her. I was also proud when the foundation she directs announced a 1.35 million dollar grant to study trans in the military. This is a prime example of the ripple effect I, and the lessons of Miss Vera's Academy, have on society, thanks to our students.

Jennifer has always been a popular name at Miss Vera's Academy, thanks in part to Jennifer Aniston and *Friends*, the most popular TV show of the '90s. Another Jennifer who will live in my heart forever is Jennifer/ James, a gentle sissy. One of my first official students, James, a self-proclaimed sissy, was totally enthusiastic about the program I established. He said, "I want to be the wind beneath your wings." And he was. Jennifer James helped put our school on the map. The story of "sissy power" was the first in our academy herstory to illustrate how self-acceptance leads to self-empowerment, and how that can empower others.

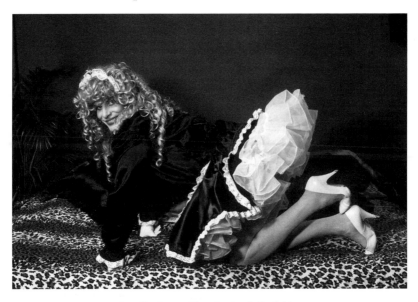

Jennifer James. Photo by Annie Sprinkle.

ЯƎWOꟼ YƧƧIƧ

MISS VERA'S FINISHING SCHOOL RECEIVED its initial publicity via a full-page story in a very influential weekly, *New York Magazine*. I had planned a party to launch the school. At the time, there were three students who asked if they could serve the party as French maids, meaning they would be transformed and wear short frilly outfits while they checked coats and served drinks and hors d'oeuvres.

I had created beautiful brochures to promote Miss Vera's Finishing School, and a friend had shown the brochure to her friend,

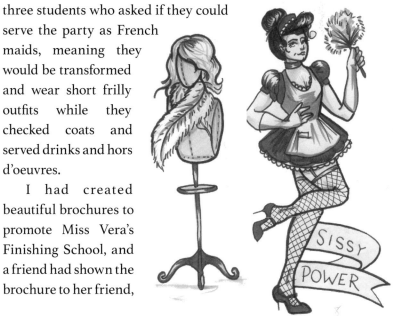

SISSY POWER

a freelance reporter named George Rush. George was intrigued by the concept of Miss Vera's. When he learned we were about to have our own coming-out party and that three of the students normally dressed in male clothes would be our serving girls, he pitched the story to *New York Magazine*. The editors loved the idea, especially if they could send a photographer.

Most of my friends and colleagues were far from camera shy, but then they were not wearing French maid uniforms. I asked the self-proclaimed sissies if they would consent to be photographed for publication. Students Jennifer and April agreed. Raquel said it was okay, but only her legs.

A couple of weeks later, the full-page story appeared. It contained photos and quotes from me, the well-known guests – Ms. Antoinette, Annie Sprinkle, Candida Royalle – and revealing comments from our three brave sissies. I said if they had been wearing camouflage and pith helmets, they could not have shown more courage under fire.

Jennifer and April empowered themselves by coming out, and us right along with them.

I lost track of Raquel and her legs.

But April transitioned soon after, the first of my students to do so. She became politically active and eventually spent much of her time being of help to others as part of an EMS team, and more recently as a life coach. That first party and press started a snowball of publicity from which many have benefited.

EXPELLED

ND THEN THERE WAS ROY, aka Mandy. More than twenty years after our founding, Mandy was the first student to be expelled from Miss Vera's Finishing School for Boys Who Want to Be Girls.

A girlfriend of Roy's encouraged him to enroll. The girlfriend lived in New York, so she came to meet me and we called Roy, who completed his application via phone.

Roy had experienced some major life changes. His mother had died the previous year. He also left the world of high-powered investments to run the business that his wife's parents had started. Roy was in his late fifties and had recently married for the second time.

At first, Roy displayed many good qualities. He had humor and enthusiasm. We decided that Mandy's very first visit would be a professional photo shoot. Roy visited websites I suggested and ordered Mandy a brand new wardrobe, her first. Most of it was in the style of a '50s television stay-at-home wife: full skirts with crinoline petticoats, like Beaver Cleaver's mom.

The deans worked their magic and transformed Roy to Mandy, using several different wigs and beautiful outfits. Mandy brought her own super-long talons for use as fingernails.

Our photographer created marvelous images. Mandy was thrilled with the results of the photo shoot. Roy was very grateful to me and the deans and asked if he might take us all out to dinner at an upscale restaurant. The deans loved the idea, so I agreed. I did, however, make one suggestion. By now, I understood that whether in Roy mode or Mandy, this student loved the spotlight and sought attention by being louder than others. I had corrected Mandy a few times. The restaurant Roy had chosen had the reputation as a place for lovers, more quiet and intimate. Plus, in a group of five or more, I always prefer a restaurant with round tables so that each guest can be part of the same conversation. I suggested to Roy that we switch to another restaurant, explaining why I thought would be a better fit for our group. Roy agreed to the change, but added that I reminded him of his ex-wife because she always wanted to change his plans. There seemed to be an attitude of belligerence in his words, and I told him that I did not want to be compared to an ex-wife. Roy said he was only joking and I didn't understand his humor. I let it drop.

That first photo shoot really shook Roy up. He loved the way he looked and felt as Mandy. "Where is this all going, Miss Vera?" he asked. I told him the point was to find out more about himself and that we could make those discoveries together. Roy took a giant step and told his wife about his visit. He showed her pictures of Mandy. His wife called me and I told her more about Miss Vera's Finishing School and the people who come here. She became supportive of Mandy. She helped her husband pick out Mandy's dress for the spring gala, Night of 1000 Gowns, our students' coming-out party.

The gala was an academy group event, but Mandy wanted everything to revolve around her schedule. I reprimanded her lightly and told her if I were to give her a report card, it would have to say, *Doesn't play well with others.*

"I've heard that since I was in second grade," was her response. She wasn't joking.

Things began to go downhill. Mandy could not accept her role as a student. She was constantly testing my authority, making jokes at my expense, and then telling me I had no sense of humor. There was an inner battle going on within Roy and Mandy, that unfortunately had begun to be further fueled by alcohol. It was not me, but one of my deans, who first used the word "misogynist" to describe this student.

Misogynist, a woman-hater. I certainly knew the term, but I wanted a more precise definition. The source I found listed a dozen ways to identify a misogynist, noting that a person might not display all of these behaviors. Roy/Mandy displayed eight of the dozen, the most telling ones being inability to accept authority from a woman and picking a particular woman as a target. The source also said this problem had usually started at an early age and, if it was never addressed, got worse. I remembered Mandy's mention of second grade and realized that I had given Roy all the help I could. Now he needed help of a different kind.

I told Roy his problem was twofold: his misogyny and his overindulgence in alcohol. I gave him the information I had found. Because I had been critical of his behavior, both as Roy and as Mandy, he chose to see me as an enemy. It was easier than taking a look at himself. Roy had been desperate to distinguish himself as a student and he succeeded: Mandy was the very first student I had ever expelled.

As difficult as it was to go through this experience with Roy, I knew I was meant to learn something from it, just as I had learned from our academy success stories. Roy and Mandy opened my eyes to the depth of anger that can lie under the surface when we explore gender roles.

Misogyny is real. Its counterpart is "misandry." Feminists are sometimes labeled man-haters by those who belittled women's fight for equal rights. But both misandry and misogyny exist. They are byproducts of living within the constraints of the gender binary.

Binary thinking supports the idea that all women behave or are supposed to behave a certain way, and the same for men. This can lead to conclusions of trust and distrust, anger as well as love. Sometimes these conclusions are conscious, sometimes unconscious.

I didn't know Roy's entire history, but I saw that he was troubled by his feelings regarding Mandy. He wanted to stay the man in charge. He needed that control. He couldn't trust himself, and he certainly couldn't trust a woman, me, or himself in a dress.

I wrote in my first book that when you start to explore gender, you may find yourself out of the closet and into Pandora's box. Whenever disenfranchised people step out to form a movement and begin to come to power, emotions that were buried rise to the surface. Frustration is often released as anger. Black power, the feminist movement, gay/lesbian/bisexual pride all demonstrate this tendency, as does the transgender movement. We blame each other when what is at fault is the outmoded system that is still in place.

In the Greek myth, Zeus gave Pandora a box as a wedding gift but told her to never open it. Pandora didn't understand why the gift came with such a rule. Try as she might, she could not stop herself from opening the box. What was released were all the ills of the world. Nasty wasps flew at Pandora and stung her all over. When she looked down into the box, she saw there was only one item left. At first, she was afraid to set it free, but then thinking nothing could be worse than what she had already experienced, she released the final item. It was Hope. Hope flew out in the form of a dragonfly. The dragonfly touched the sores left by the wasps and healed them. Pandora had released pain and suffering, but she had also allowed Hope to follow.

What you find when you begin to explore your cross gender options may open up fear and frustration. But once you feel and acknowledge these emotions, you can begin to examine them. You can take action: accept what you want, make changes that you need. Fear and frustration can no longer hold sway over you. Instead, you can feel renewed love of yourself and in others.

Cross Gender Fun for All

LIFE AS ART LIFE AS ART

MY SCHOOL AND I HAVE HELPED to change the face and the figure of society. We've made discoveries by encouraging new ways of being. I've said I am in the business of making dreams come true, but this is not so much a business as an art. I encourage you, as you create your cross-gender icon, to think of yourself as an artist of life.

In 2014, I received a grant from the Franklin Furnace in support of my work in the field of performance art. Performance art involves the body of the artist and is presented to an audience in a dramatic way,

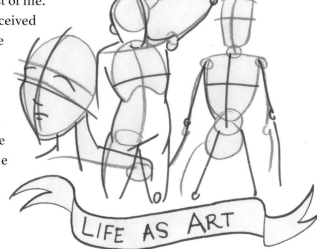

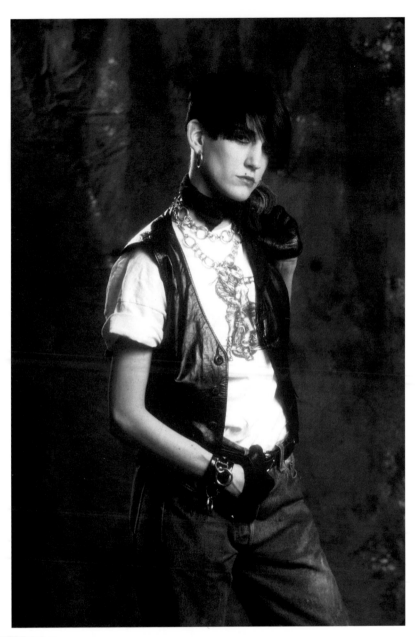

Trash in denim. Photo by Annie Sprinkle.

Cross Gender Fun for All

but unlike a play, it does not follow a script, nor does it need to take place on a formal stage. Performance art is full of surprises.

Franklin Furnace was created by artist Martha Wilson. It is an incubator of performance art and has supported the work of such bold artists as Karen Finley, Tim Miller, Holly Hughes, John Fleck – the controversial "NEA Four" who were criticized by those who thought the National Endowment for the Arts should not fund art that was dangerous to the status quo.

In Martha's own work, she has presented herself as a woman in many different roles or types: goddess, working girl, earth mother, lesbian. More specifically, she's presented as Bill Clinton and Barbara Bush, perhaps her most well-known personae. If only Martha Wilson had actually been U.S. First Lady, what a wonderful world this would be! In any case, she is "first lady of performance art."

Recently, I discussed this book with the great sex educator Dr. Betty Dodson, known for her books on liberating masturbation and sexual empowerment. Betty said she was at first confused by the term "gender," but now understood that what we call "gender" today was referred to as "sex roles" in the '50s and '60s when she began her professional life. She showed me the cover of her memoir *My Romantic Love Wars,* which bears the photo of a gorgeous blonde office type, hair pulled back in a tight bun, horn-rimmed glasses. "No one gets that this was me," she exclaimed. Indeed, the Betty on the cover looks very unlike the Betty of today. And it's not about age. The Betty on the cover was working on Madison Avenue at 20, with plans to be a fashion illustrator. Just a few years later, that young Betty moved to San Francisco and wore a short butch haircut, leather shorts and combat boots in the new role she described as "the tough little dyke."

"There was a time I wore a long robe trimmed in gold and my head was nearly shaved clean. People didn't know whether I was male or female. They didn't know what to make of me, but they cleared a path for me as I moved through a room. It was a look that commanded respect."

Betty has played with gender throughout her life. She just called it by another term. Sex and gender used to be thought of as the same word. But gender is a role or roles, gender is performance.

My personal mentor is Linda Montano, whose motto is "Life is Art." In my previous books and during on-campus lessons, I have always encouraged Miss Vera's academy students to think of their transgender explorations as performance art. This is a dynamic experience. The make-up and wardrobe, walking and voice, all aspects of presentation, aid in your performance. The use of those outer trappings to reveal the unseen truth of feelings and emotions are what turn the performance into art.

Taking your art in into the street, sharing it with others, gives your art life. The great thing about being an artist is that it gives you license to take risks. The rewards of those risks can fulfill your dreams.

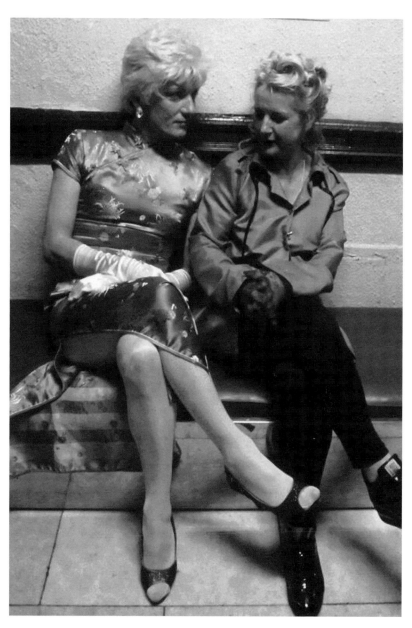

A happy couple of graduates. Photo by Linda Troeller.

Cross Gender Fun for All

THE GREAT TRANSFORMERS

THE GREAT TRANSFORMERS

THERE WAS A TIME before the emergence of Caitlyn Jenner, a time I refer to as "Trans BC." During that time there were people who facilitated others in transformation, who were guides to those who wanted to take those

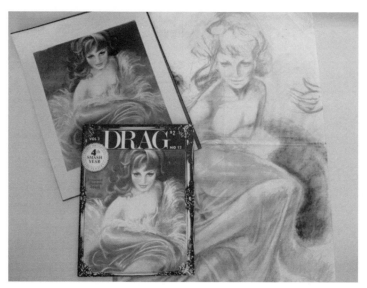

Lee Brewster's Drag Mag. Art by Vicky West. Courtesy Mariette Pathy Allen.

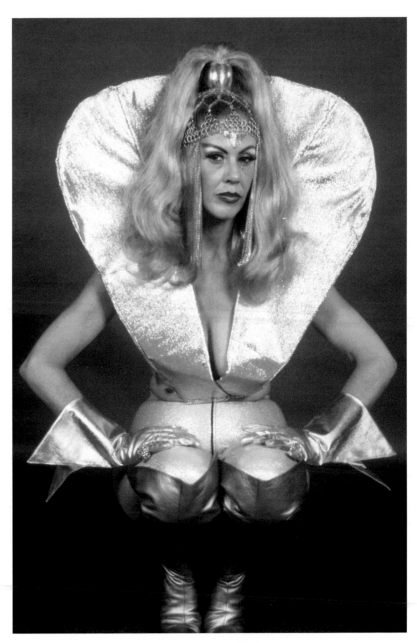

Ms. Antoinette. Photo by Zorro.

Cross Gender Fun for All

artistic risks. Not all them identified as artists themselves, but they were. Here are some who have influenced me.

Meeting Annie Sprinkle was particularly momentous for me. She became not only a best friend, but a guide. Annie Sprinkle is a catalyst with an amazing ability to bring people together. Annie is a transformer herself. Some examples of her work in this field are "Sluts and Goddesses" – the workshop and then the video that encourages women to explore these aspects of themselves. In the field of gender, Annie and her romantic partner at the time created "Linda, Les and Annie: The First Female to Male Transsexual Love Story."

It was through Annie that I met other great transformers. The first was Ms. Antoinette, she of the leather catsuit and six-inch stiletto boots. I met Antoinette in about 1980 when she was a special guest at "the Sprinkle Salon." Then I spent a summer with her in Orange County, California, where she published *Reflections*, which described itself as "the magazine devoted to the exotic lifestyle" – in this case, bondage, discipline, dominance and submission. Her husband, Dick, a doctor, aka "Master Zorro," was the magazine's photographer and, later, videographer. Antoinette's love of fashion inspired her to dress the part of the dominatrix as well as to create an entire clothing line so that other women, men and those who identified as transvestites could explore their fantasies.

A leather catsuit might better be called dressing "cross-species," inspiring on many several levels. For Antoinette and others, it would be as powerful as the finest pinstripe suit. Later, her fabric of choice would be the shiny plastic, polyvinyl chloride, and she became the queen of PVC.

Antoinette's assistant was Reb Stout. Reb created three female and three male alteregos. He had originally come to Antoinette after years as a violent biker. Reb once said that had he not let himself explore gender play, he would have wound up in jail, or "dead in a gutter," he had gotten into so many fights.

The kind of dressing represented by Antoinette, Reb and also by some gender explorers is referred to as "fetish dressing." All clothing is significant in some way other than protective garb, but often clothing – because of the way if feels or smells, and/or the memories it recalls – is referred to as fetish dressing.

Fetish clothing is about sexuality and power, but also about perception: how you perceive yourself and how others perceive you. You can imbue any article of clothing with more power. Perhaps you are someone who has held on to the clothing of a loved one who has passed, or a young woman who loves to sleep in her boyfriend's t-shirt. Certain fabrics such as leather and latex are more obvious in their sensual content: wearing them can actually make your temperature rise, make you wet. Corsets and high heels manipulate the body in ways that are hard to ignore: the corset is a firm embrace and for a moment can leave you breathless; high heels raise the buttocks to provocative heights.

When I arrived at their home, what I have referred to as "the chambers of Ms. Antoinette," she sized up my appearance, my sundress and make-up free face, and said, "Oh, I see. You are a *natural girl*." There was a certain disdain in her voice.

Two months later, I returned to New York twenty pounds thinner, thanks to Dr. Dick's diet plan. I wore a skin-tight spandex dress with a slit up the side, designed by Antoinette, and spike heels. My fingernails were bejeweled talons. I remember feeling all eyes on me as I crossed the street at Union Square on my way to an appointment. I'd never felt more the *femme fatale*.

Not only had Antoinette provided me with an education about fetish clothing in general, I learned about the effect clothing specifically designed to turn me into a sexpot had on me. Later, I brought those lessons into my Academy.

Not long after, on a return visit to New York, I went with Antoinette to visit Lee's Mardi Gras, the famous transvestite boutique. Today, cross-gender explorations are recognized as an art form, but not very long ago gender play was against the law. One who helped change the law was another great transformer I was privileged to know and love, Mr. Lee Brewster.

Lee's Mardi Gras was actually a 5000-square-foot department store that catered to the needs of male to female cross-dressers. It had existed at various locations from 1969 until Lee's death in 2001. The business was a creative work of art, from a former party hostess who was a political activist.

Upon arriving in New York City from West Virginia, where he had worked as a clerk for the FBI, Lee became involved with the Mattachine Society, an early gay rights organization. Lee was a fantastic host and he soon became director of the group's social events. Lee also loved to dress in boas, heels and gowns, and when the Mattachines decided cross-dressing would not be permitted at their events, Lee decided to throw his own parties, which then became infamous.

Lee's parties were a haven for cross-dressers of every persuasion. They were open events and all kinds of celebrities came. Shirley MacLaine was among those who attended the very last one. Lee published a newsletter which became *Drag Magazine,* with lush illustrations by Vicky West. Eventually partygoers began coming to Lee to find shopping resources.

Lee's Mardi Gras boutique began as a sideline in Lee's apartment. From his vantage point, Lee understood that he was part of a vast community whose civil rights were denied. It was still possible to be arrested for being gay or lesbian or for dressing in drag. So Lee, along with others, formed The Queens Liberation Front that helped eliminate oppressive city ordinances.

When I began Miss Vera's Finishing School, I was continuing the work of these and other pioneers. I

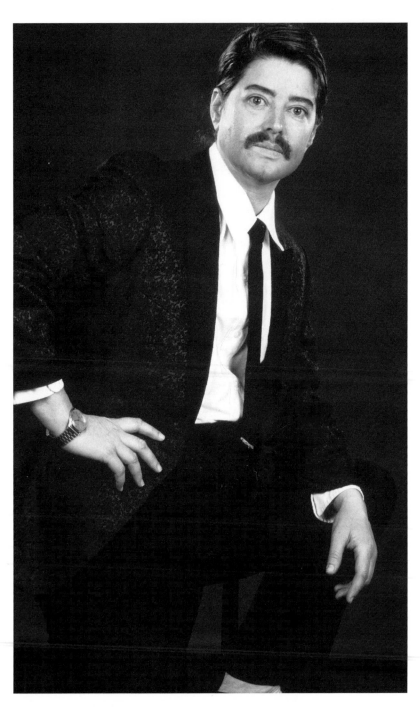

Diane Torr as Danny King. Photo by Annie Sprinkle.

Cross Gender Fun for All

took courage in the fact that Lee's Mardi Gras boutique existed. Not only could I bring my students there to shop, Lee always gave me permission to bring the media with me, as long as they respected the privacy of his clients.

The closest I ever got to my own physical female to male transformation occurred circa 1989 under the tutelage of Johnny Science. Johnny had been born Susan and Susan had been dressing as a boy and transforming girls into guys from a very early age. As Johnny, he founded what he named an "F2M" (female to male) fraternity that met regularly at the home of his friend Katherine "Kit" Racklin. Kit is now a leading psychologist whose specialty is transgender.

It was Annie who invited me to attend an F2M gathering with her. The meetings were fun social events. Johnny was a terrific performer. He'd had his own band, called "Science."

Johnny was asked to host an evening at the Limelight night club. He offered to transform me and other women for the event. I slicked back my hair and Johnny gave me a goatee, coupled with a heavy dose of 5 o'clock shadow, but I still wore a dress – so the result was more that of a bearded lady than a gent. I couldn't get away from wearing a dress, but my new swarthy appearance imbued me with confidence. I did not care about living up to standards of beauty, I felt perfect in my own strangeness.

I wrote about the experience in "Veronica Vera's New York," a monthly column that appeared in *ADAM,* an adult magazine. Annie, too, had a column in *ADAM,* and a few months earlier had chosen Johnny as an interview subject. To illustrate her interview, she needed someone who would be transformed female to male by Johnny. Diane Torr was recommended and Annie hired Diane. This brought Johnny and Diane together for the first time, and the collaboration was perfect.

Diane Torr had arrived in New York in 1976 from England after completing studies in theatre, dance, music and creative writing. Her desire was to establish herself as a New York based artist. Her early dance performances in New York received excellent reviews and in 1982 she began exploring gender as a subject in *Arousing*

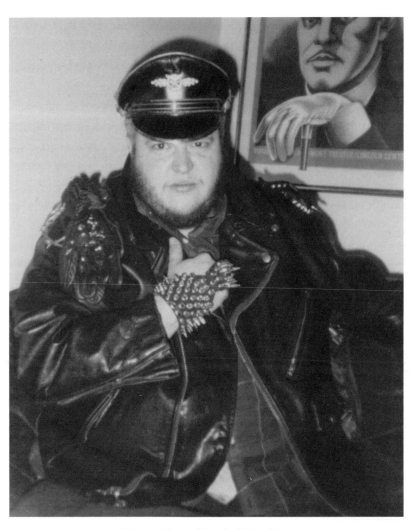

Johnny Science. Photo by Kit Rachlin.

Reconstructions, with visual artist Bradley Wester. Like so many significant moments in crossgender history, this performance was documented by photographer Mariette Pathy Allen.

In addition to dance and theater pieces, Diane performed various male characters in clubs: TR3, Mudd Club, Danceteria, CBGB Gallery. It was mainly in the Pyramid Club that Diane's performances in male drag received a particularly enthusiastic response. Artist Shelly Mars also regularly performed her male drag personas at Pyramid. Pyramid was also home to Lady Bunny, Linda Simpson and others who would create Wigstock.

Following that photo shoot in 1989, Diane participated in Johnny Science's 3 hour workshop for which Johnny coined the term "Drag King." Johnny's expertise was in make-up. Visually, his drag kings were very convincing portraits. He knew how to bind the breasts and how to "pack" a penis, but he had no theater training. Diane told Johnny if he was going to create a workshop he needed to include physical exercises, scene studies and more. They decided to work together giving the "Drag King Workshops." Johnny did all of the make-up, and Diane facilitated the character development of all of the participants.

Coincidentally, it was in 1989 that I first supervised the education and transformation of "Sally Sissy Ribbons," the first student in what I would soon call Miss Vera's Finishing School for Boys Who Want to Be Girls. Both my academy and Johnny and Diane's Drag King Workshops received lots of media attention throughout the '90s.

The publications and cross-dressing galas of Lee Brewster, the magazines and "Dress to Thrill" fetish dress parties of Ms. Antoinette, the aboveground recognition of Miss Vera's Finishing School and Johnny and Diane's Workshops all had a political element. Diane remembers how she and Johnny punched the air with their fists when they heard the phrase "drag king" on television for the first time. All were changing the status quo.

Eventually, Johnny's activism as well as his personal exploits wore him thin, but Diane continued, for a while in New York and then in Europe. Diane felt the New York drag king scene had become too formulaic, just make-up and lip-synching in bars. In Europe she continued to develop her own performances as well as the workshop. She changed the workshop name to "Man For a Day."

Today, Diane Torr's "Man For A Day" workshops are held around the world. The film "Man For A Day" by Katrina Peters documents a weekend-long workshop that Diane led in Berlin. At the end of the weekend, the film shows that each of the women has been empowered in some unexpected way. Though none went into the workshop with a particular agenda, there have been real life changes.

One particularly convincing participant actually went to a car dealership and used her male guise as a means to cut a deal that she thought would have been unthinkable as a woman. Another made a career change to honor her political ambitions. An important distinction to the workshop is that the intention is not to "pass," but rather to question what is considered a given.

Similarly, at Miss Vera's Finishing School, the goal is not simply transformation but integration, to take what you learn in your cross-gender identity and incorporate into your life, to give you more options.

"We're all born naked, the rest is drag" is a quote from RuPaul, a great transformer who brought drag queen performance to the masses via television and *RuPaul's Drag Race*. RuPaul's contributions include great imagination, humor and most of all, great heart. "Love" is the most prominent word in RuPaul's vocabulary.

We've come a long way from naked, and a long way from the time when the first purpose of clothing was to keep us warm. When clothing became fashion it took on political implications. It became a means of self-expression. It could be a source of liberation, but could also be used to confine. In both Eastern and Western cultures, sumptuary laws came into existence. These statutes were designed to regulate behavior and maintain status quo. In ancient Greece, a woman could not go out in an embroidered robe unless she was a prostitute. In Rome, the number of stripes on a man's tunic was regulated by his social rank. In China and Japan, sumptuary laws existed around burials and armaments. The Islamic laws that center on clothing are many: gold jewelry on men is forbidden, for example, while on women it is encouraged. The tradition of the burkha lives on in some Muslim countries.

Many of these sumptuary laws have disappeared. Some were never that strong to begin with. Yet the idea of clothing as a symbol persists.

We will put those symbols to use as our tools – better yet, as our toys, something to pull from the big dress-up box. So, let's play.

YOUR ENROLLMENT APPLICATION

YOUR ENROLLMENT APPLICATION

WHETHER OR NOT YOU actually visit Miss Vera's Finishing School, the enrollment application is an essential first step. We need your responses in order to design a program for you. These questions will help you think about what you want and need to give your life more balance. The action of completing the application is a "declaration" of your needs. Completing the application is a sign of cooperation: you are ready to follow instructions and proceed.

Starting Gender _____   Cross Gender _____

Your Current Name _____   Proposed Name _____

Present Age _____ Cross Gender Age_____

Marital Status_____

Measurements: (actual)

Height _____

Weight _____

Chest/Breast_____

Waist _____

Hips _____

Shoe size_____

What qualities would you like to nurture or enhance?

How do you envision your cross gender self?

Who are your cross gender role models?

Full body Transformation?_____ Iconic symbol?_____ Undecided?_____

Guide to Completing Your Enrollment Application

1. **Your Gender:** Your current gender or the one in which you've lived most of your life; and your cross-gender opposite, the one you are moving toward.

   This is not a trick question, though it may seem to be. On the one hand, I've stated that the gender binary is over: masculine and feminine are not enough. These were fragile categories to begin with. In the days when human survival was dependent on populating the planet, binary gender held sway. It was essential that female and males recognize each other and mate. But with scientific and social advancement, there was more recognition that, except for the needs of procreation, a gender binary was an artificial construct.

   Now we recognize a third gender, transgender. It's my belief that the essence of humanity is trans, the breath within each of us is gender neutral or gender fluid. It was a complex combination of nature and nurture that made us think that our roles in life offered only two options.

   For our purposes we are going to work from what we know as the gender binary to become more gender-fluid or trans. If you already identify as a trans person, you can still use this process to access or enhance certain qualities.

2. **Your name:** The one you write at the beginning of this process is likely to change by the end. Choosing a new name for your cross gender self is like giving yourself a new birth certificate. Use your imagination. What's in a name? It can be plenty.

I want you to really get to know your cross gender icon. To be on a first-name basis, you've got to give your icon a name. This familiarity will make this part of you more real – and the more real your icon feels, the more you can believe in the qualities your icon brings to you. You might choose a name that pays homage to a role model or a particular quality. I chose the name Vera as my pen name because Vera means "true" and I wanted to write the truth as I understood my truth to be. In choosing a name for my icon, I thought about the name Stuart in honor of my husband Stuart, but with a slightly different spelling because I think as humans we all have the responsibility to be stewards of our gifts: our talents, our planet, our families. I hope to be a good steward, or Stewart.

Or perhaps I'll be Ares, the messenger. I've got plenty to say, lots of messages to impart.

Or simply, Señor! It's got a certain gravitas. Señor will also help me age gracefully. Hmmm, Señor it is!

Many academy students feminize their male names. Steve is Stephanie; Jeff is Jennifer. Female to male Samantha could be Sam; Lisa could be Leon. Or pick a name that refers to a quality or occupation. "Eric" means "king forever." "Brianna" is "noble one." "Andrew" means "virile" or "manly." "Mabel" translates to "adorable."

3. **Your age:** It's a tiny word, just three letters, but a word that carries so much significance. They used to say you only live once, but these days there are many who would argue. In the virtual world, people live many lives – and so can you, as you create your cross-gender self. You can stay the same age to simply "see how the other half lives." Just as your name may change, so can you change your age, in either direction. Recapture the daring spirit of youth, or align yourself with the wisdom of years.

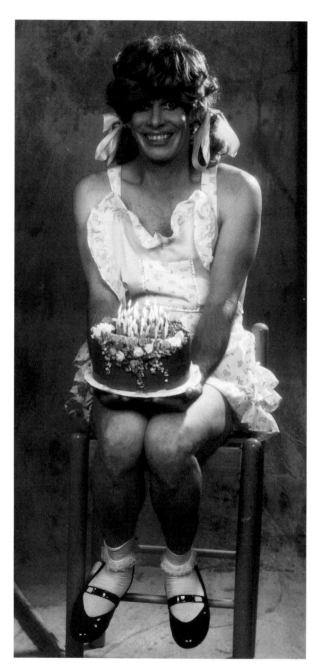

Happy Birthday Jennifer James. Photo by Annie Sprinkle.

I said the gender binary held sway when it was necessary for survival. Now just the opposite is true. Cross gender play can add to longevity.

4. **Marital status:** Will you be engaged in this process as an individual, or as part of a couple? Either way, the benefits are tremendous. Role play is a way in which couples spice up a relationship but it can also be a way in which you reach new levels of understanding and communication. Talk therapy is fine, but clothing and props can help you and a partner step out of yourselves, leaving egos behind, to learn and relate in less threatening, more playful ways.

5. **Measurements.** Use a tape measure for accuracy. You can do this alone, or ask a friend to help. We'll start with your actual frame as the armature, then use clothing, prosthetics, make-up and tape to add or subtract as needed and sculpt the new you. The creation of your cross-gender icon may involve only the tiniest change: polish one fingernail if you are going male to female; remove your polish and cut those nails short, to go from female to male. You may not need a full set of clothes, but it's best to be prepared. Plus it's nice for me to have some idea of the physical you.

6. **Your Goals.** What are the qualities you would like to enhance?

   Life is energy and energy can be either kinetic or moving; or potential, at rest.

   If you are creating a male icon, choose qualities from the list on the left. If, creating a female icon, choose from the list on the right. Feel free to add qualities you think I may have overlooked.

Masculine _____   Feminine _____

Logical_____   Intuitive _____

Strong_____   Fragile _____

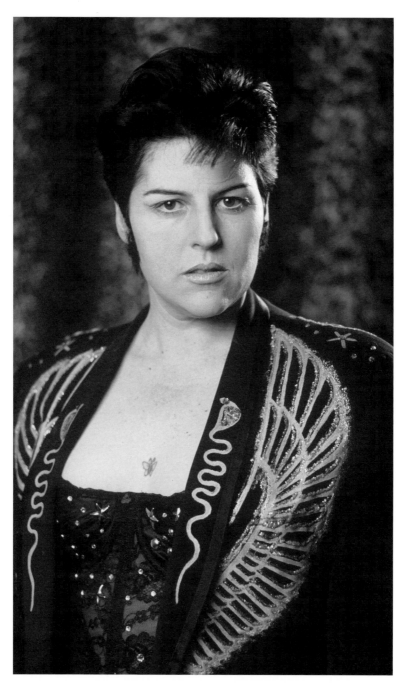

Leslie Lowe as Elvis. Photo by Annie Sprinkle.

Hard Working _____ Playful _____

Virile _____ Fertile/Sexy _____

Stoic _____ Emotional _____

Leader _____ Follower/supporter _____

Protector _____ Nurturer _____

Dominant _____ Submissive _____

Hunter _____ Homemaker _____

Active _____ Passive _____

Dynamic _____ Thoughtful _____

Builder _____ Decorator _____

Confident _____ Desirable _____

Detached _____ Compassionate _____

Aloof _____ Sociable _____

Financier _____ Shopper _____

The ones on the left are traditionally thought of as masculine, while those on the right are those traditionally thought of as feminine. This is because society since time immemorial has been based on archetypes, which are actually methods of function. They populate our myths and stories and are part of our collective unconscious.

Originally, performance of these functions was based on instinct and the basic physical reality. The male of the species was physically stronger, the female was fertile, the life carrier. In order to survive, the stronger male had to protect the childbearing female. He had a job to perform and he

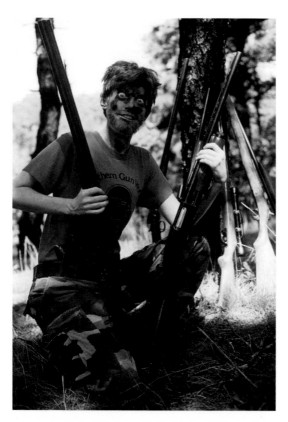

Katharine as Billy Joe Freeman. Photo by Annie Sprinkle.

needed to be efficient. To be efficient, man used logic. While male logic would say, only the strong survive, the female understood that every child had something to offer.

The role of woman was to bear and nurture children. In order to inspire the man to participate in conception she used eros to attract his attention: a wiggle of her comely buttocks was a potent signal.

The basic male archetypes or roles, as seen throughout our stories, are king, warrior, magician and lover. The basic female archetypes are queen, mother, wise woman and lover. All of the jobs that we have in society can be connected to these archetypes.

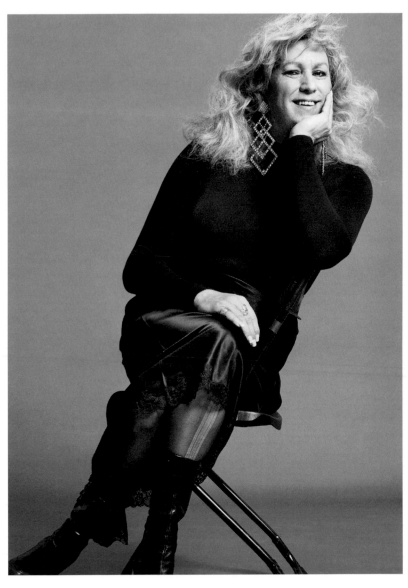

Karlie. Photo by Philippe Vogelenzang.

Political leaders and CEOs are kings and queens. Firemen, policemen and soldiers are warriors, but so are mothers. Priests, gurus, scientists and artists are magicians.

Cross Gender Fun for All

As you've grown, you've probably been socialized to accentuate certain traits according to the gender binary. Women accentuate feminine traits, men accentuate male traits. Our survival no longer depends on strict adherence to the gender binary, nor has it for centuries. You have the potential to own and display any of the traits on these lists.

Throughout the history of civilization, there have been numerous big shifts that have affected humans. An early one was the move from being dependent on hunting to farming; the creation of cities, the industrial revolution... the Internet. Societal advances such as medical discoveries leading to longer lives, universal education, technological advances gave humans new options and inspired us to escape proscribed roles and look for more opportunities for pleasure, growth and fulfillment.

The individuals who visit my academy are a reflection of this desire – as, to some extent, is everyone who is transgender. There is a term in biology that describes the harmony within which our bodies function and stay regulated and stable. This term is "homeostasis," and it can refer to the mind as well as the body. Psychologists use the term homeostasis to describe when individual psyches are in balance. We have arrived at a time when men and women recognize the need to live authentic hybrid lives. We are in an amazing place in terms of human evolution, and it is important to understand that we are all in it together.

7. **Archetypes/Stereotypes/Shadows.** How do you envision your cross gender self? At Miss Vera's Finishing School, the process of creating your cross gender self is collaboration. We are not taking an idea and imposing our idea on you. We are working together to reveal and support qualities and talents you would like to enhance. It's important that you are aware and conscious of your participation.

The original application which I designed for trans-feminine students provided some suggestions: sissy maid, sexy vamp, whorish slut, young wife, model, sophisticated career woman, mommy's little girl, pregnant, conservative librarian, other... This list drew adverse criticism from some feminists, particularly academics, who said that I was encouraging female stereotypes. What the critics failed to understand was that it was students – who spent their lives enmeshed in the male persona – who wanted to achieve this balance. These suggestions are points of access on the path to the great female archetype in all her aspects: queen, mother, wise woman, lover...

Had they been born in ancient Greece, these students might have devoted themselves to different goddesses at different times: the sexy vamps, whorish sluts, and young wives to Aphrodite, goddess of love; sophisticated career women and conservative librarians to Athena for wisdom, and to Artemis for courage and adventure. My instructions to the student were that he could pick one description of his femmeself, or more than one. Those who picked one usually chose sexy vamp/whorish slut or sophisticated career woman.

Identifying their feelings as erotic made sense since the anima, the inner female in every man, is aligned with Eros. In picking the description "sophisticated career woman," the fellows often chose what they saw as the flip side of their lives as men. It would not be unusual for a someone crossing from female to male to pick the description "corporate honcho" or "statesman," because that coincides with the animus being aligned with logic and practicality.

I cannot emphasize enough how the goal of this cross gender exploration is not simply transformation but integration. As you cross gender borders, whether for a day or a lifetime, I don't want or expect you to forget all of the qualities that serve you well in your original gender. "Don't throw the baby out with the bath water," as they say. The goal is to take what you learn in your cross-gender role and integrate it into your persona so that you have a richer, fuller life. Some of your original traits can benefit from a new balance, other traits might best be eliminated and replaced with others.

A cross gender exploration can be a bit treacherous. Sometimes we create a cross gender persona that is not very evolved and simply not likable. For that reason it is good to have a guide to help you, or to do this gender play with a partner who can give you feedback. Etiquette classes are included in the curriculum at Miss Vera's Finishing School, for this and other reasons. People think of etiquette as table manners, but etiquette is really about treating others with the care and respect we wish to be treated ourselves.

We all have preconceived notions and attitudes about persons of the opposite gender. A woman might discover that the first male persona she puts on is that of a "macho pig." A man might begin the exploration of his inner femme as a "nasty bitch." It's a start, but you're not finished. That's why you're in school. You owe it to yourself and to society to go further.

8. **Who are your cross gender role models?** Who do you admire and want to emulate? This can be someone real or an imaginary character; someone famous or someone known only to you and your inner circle; someone living or dead. It may be easier to choose a role model from someone whom you know but who has died. A person's good qualities can be more outstanding when they are no longer around to make mistakes. Pick one person, or more than one.

You might pick someone because of the way that person looks, but I suggest you give it more thought. It's likely even if you are picking someone because of their physical appearance, they have other qualities that enhance the way they look. Those inner qualities are what make them really

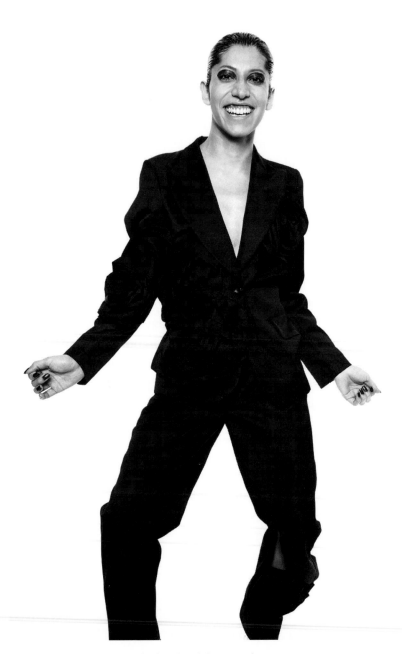

Eriel. Photo by Philippe Vogelenzang.

Cross Gender Fun for All

outstanding. Of course, there are others whose looks can go from splendid to scary if they don't have the admirable traits to match that first impression. So choose wisely. Picking a role model will also help you to pinpoint the qualities or talents that you want to nurture in yourself. It's wonderful to have heroes and sheroes.

9. **Decision to move forward.** Now that you have a better idea of what is involved in this process, are you ready to decide how you would like to proceed? Will you opt for a full physical transformation, or make a small change... or perhaps, start off with a small change and then take a bigger step?

PART TWO

FULL BODY PHYSICAL TRANSFORMATION

A S AN ACTOR USES MAKE-UP, props and coaching to get into a new role, so we use these same methods at Miss Vera's Finishing School to help you create your cross gender self. The difference between you and an actor in a play is that you – not some outside author – are involved in the creating of your character, and you will continue to use many qualities of this new persona in your everyday life.

Once we've built the form, the functions follow. Your cross gender self will learn to walk and talk, and will discover talents and aspects of personality that have lain dormant. These props and lessons of behavior modification are tools that we use to kickstart your process.

The Internet is a wealth of very useful and very detailed information. It's not my purpose to impart information here that you can acquire much more thoroughly in step-by-step videos via YouTube. But I will share some of the most significant steps and tricks of the trade. These work, and they are fun.

Our goal is not simply transformation but integration, so no matter how you self-identify you have unfettered access to your full range of options. With freedom of expression, whatever your

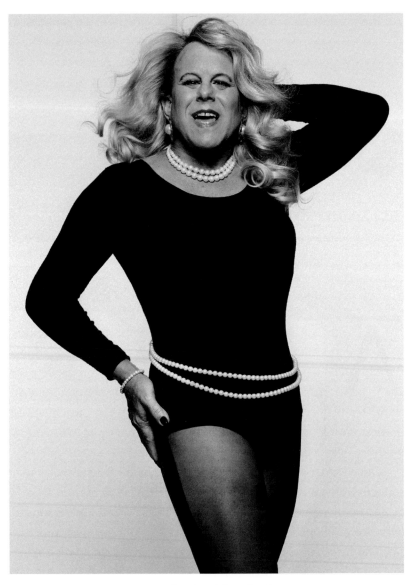

Rita Renner. Photo by Philippe Vogelenzang.

fashion statement, you will be a happier, healthier, sexier human being. In whatever gender we humans present, trans is our inner life.

Your physical design depends on morphology, projection and function. Morphology means the body that you have; projection means the image of the man or woman you want to convey. Function means activity – will you simply pose, or perform?

PHYSICAL DESIGN: THE MAJOR DIFFERENCES

A sperm is a hard worker, a swimmer, task oriented; the egg floats and invites the sperm to her. From these beginnings, activity vs attraction, all else has followed. Here are some of the most typical physical differences when comparing women and men. This will be a helpful guide in creating your cross gender icon, particularly if you do not have a specific role model, but just want to let your new form guide your new function.

FIGURE

Women's bodies are soft and curvy. Men's bodies are hard and straight.

Not every woman has an hourglass figure, but that is the classic form, so we'll start there. The hourglass means that her breasts and hips are equal or nearly equal in measurement and her waistline is about ten inches smaller.

The typical male figure is broadest at the chest; his waist measures about the same as his hips and that measurement is about ten inches smaller than his chest.

To go from male to female, we'll add padding and prosthetics to create a bosom and fuller buttocks. A corset would help build a waistline, and if a corset is used there could be less need for hip pads.

To go from female to male, you might still use padding, but put it in the shoulders to give a broader chest and downplay the bosom. Loose clothing helps camouflage curves. Elasticized bandages such as ACE bandages can be used to bind the breasts and flatten the chest. A tight-fitting sports bra could also do the trick.

Short-term options for adding curves: breast forms made of silicone and a variety of materials, padded panties, full body suits.

More long-term options for adding or subtracting: diet, exercise, hormones, surgery.

BODY HAIR

Women have less. If you are going from male to female, subtract body hair.

Men have more. If you are going from female to male, add body hair.

My academy students have always complained that shaving the face is a ritual they hate. But aside from the hair atop their heads, they would happily remove every other hair on their bodies. Less body hair means that you feel everything more, especially the soft silky fabric of your feminine clothes.

To go from female to male, a woman will add more facial hair. The easiest way to do this will be with make-up, creating a five o'clock shadow. If you want to get really macho, snip off some pubic hair and glue it to your chest. Body hair is such a sign of manliness, whether going from male to female, or female to male, the change in body hair has a dramatic effect. And that's exactly what we want.

Short-term removal: shaving, waxing.

Long-term removal: electrolysis, laser, female hormones.

Short-term addition: make-up, false mustaches and beards.

Long-term addition: male hormones.

WIGS, MUSTACHES AND BEARDS

Male to female, choose longer locks.

Female to male, choose a shorter look.

From male to female: Long cascading locks make you feel feminine. We choose wigs that complement the shape of your face, but we also respect that you may have a specific image you want to project, so that may affect the wig we ultimately choose. A recent male to female student looked great in a short bob for daytime, but when that student wanted to feel sexier, we chose long platinum tresses to complement her lingerie.

There are synthetic and human hair wigs. You can find inexpensive and expensive styles in both types. A cheaper wig will have less hair. Take a look at the back of the wig. If you can see the weave

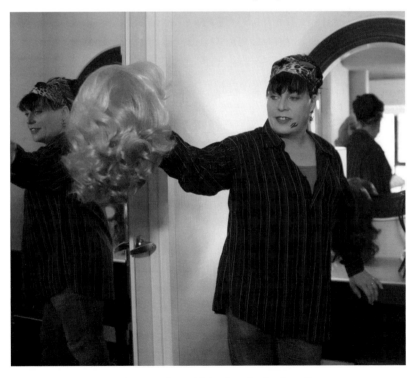

Miss Shannon, dean of 'do's. Photo by Daphne Chan.

that holds it together, that is because the hair is thinner, so don't expect a long life out of that 'do. A wig called "monofilament" has a sort of built-in scalp at the top, which makes it more breathable and more comfortable, definitely a plus. A lace-front wig gives you a natural hairline. This is a very realistic look, because it looks like the hair is growing right out of your head and it doesn't need bangs. Lace-fronts used to be much more expensive but now there are many more economical versions. Thank you, China.

If you're going from female to male, you probably have more hair to play with than a man who wants to create a feminine appearance. There are wigs in men's styles, but there are not nearly as many to choose from as feminine styles and they tend to be more expensive. My friend Diane Torr advises women in her "Man For A Day" workshop to forgo a wig, and don't stuff it all up into a hat. Just use your normal hair to create a masculine look. If you don't want to cut long hair, pull it back in a low ponytail, gathered at the nape of your neck, not in the middle of your scalp. Another option would be to use gel to slick back your hair and tame curls. Hair gel will be very helpful to create a more masculine style, no matter what your normal length.

Long hair is still considered more feminine, but there are some long-haired styles that are more gender neutral. Long flowing locks are worn by hippie guys as well as New Age gurus and more spiritual types. Long hair on a man can be very romantic, so if your male role model is Fabio, no need to clip those curls. Another long-haired style that works for women too is to pull up the hair that is normally around the face and secure it at the crown, but let the rest of the hair hang down. On a man it's a very casual, even a slacker look. Jeff Bridges has carried it off. Once you have your male hair style, if you would like to accentuate it with a chapeau, I won't say no.

If you want to have more fun with facial hair, add a mustache or beard. This can definitely take you one step further from your daily self. But remember, these items have personalities. Again, you need to consider the shape of your face and the image you want to project. There's a fine line between Tom Selleck and Groucho Marx, but then, if Groucho is your role model, more power to you!

HAIRDOS

Short-term addition: Wigs.

Short-term removal: Haircut, hair gel, tie backs.

Long-term addition: Hair systems, letting it grow.

GENITALIA

Women: Hidden

Men: Prominent

Here's the fun part, adding and subtracting the penis. The area between a woman's thighs is smooth and flat, while the penis of a man causes a bulge. To go from female to male, a woman packs her own.

A penis can be constructed by filling a condom with cotton. You can make it any size you want. The average penis is a bit over six inches, so you decide how cocky you want to be. You can also use a

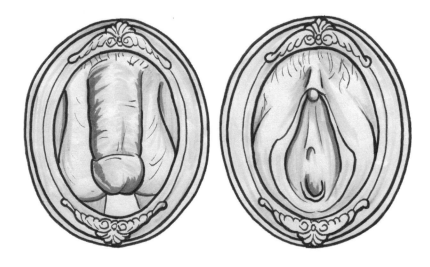

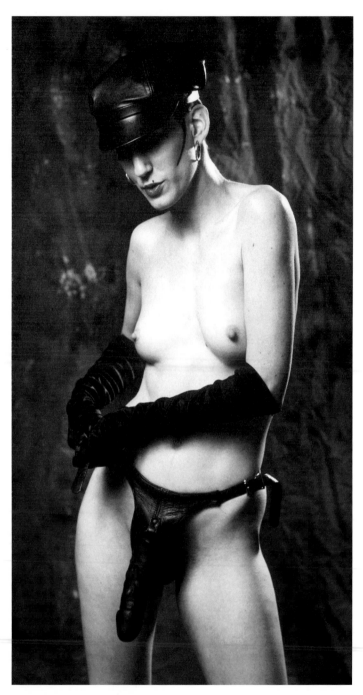

Trash with strap-on. Photo by Annie Sprinkle.

strap-on dildo and harness. This will come in very handy when we discuss your options for your cross gender sex life. As I said at the start, you don't have to do a full transformation to create a cross gender icon, you can just make a tiny change as a reminder. But if you're creating a full portrait of a man, don't skip the dick.

The tried and true way to hide a penis is to tuck. The most effective way is to use the skin of your scrotal sac as layaway storage for your testicles. Believe, it or not, they will fit nicely inside. Then pull your penis downward. A tight panty called a gaff will hold your penis in place. If you don't want to tuck, then wear a full skirt, preferably with lots of petticoats.

Long-term options for adding or subtracting genitalia: surgery.

SURGICAL OPTIONS

Nothing happens in a vacuum. The end of the gender binary, which we are experiencing now, is directly related to our awareness of the transgender phenomenon. Advances and events in other fields have influenced the growth of our transgender population. Among the influences, two of prime importance are 1) medical advances in plastic surgery and hormones, which give people the bodies that match their true identities; and 2) the Internet, which allows for information sharing and support among like-minded people.

If you have a desire to make a permanent change in your gender presentation, you will find a lot of plastic surgeons gathered at any of the transgender conferences that take place in different cities across the country. Many of the group workshops are presented by doctors who outline their procedures with careful detail. They are also available for free individual consults, and in the banquet room their tables are often filled with current and former patients who model that doctor's skill. Some plastic surgeons specialize in one particular area, such as facial feminization or masculinization, or genital congruency. Others build clinics that offer a wide variety of change.

The availability of such experts has greatly reduced the fear and mystery associated with these procedures. This familiarity with trans-related surgeries mirrors society's general change in attitude regarding plastic surgery. Whether plastic surgery is deemed necessary or cosmetic, we as a society are much more open to it.

It's not so far-fetched to envision a time in the near future when shopping malls might offer "Body Parts Emporiums" where you could choose from a selection of options: new nose, eye lift, breasts (on or off), penis, vagina and vulva, facial feminization and on and on. Hormone cocktails served in the waiting room.

MAKE-UP

"Make-up" refers to a whole group of items that you can use to change or enhance your appearance, particularly facial appearance. The term is a perfect description of the action, for these make-up items help create the new you. If you are going from male to female, use make-up to re-sculpt your face. If you are going from female to male, it is the absence of make-up that can make a huge difference.

Professionals are called make-up "artists," because whether the canvas is on a face or in a frame, the principles are the same. Light areas stand out, dark areas recede. There are many books and many, many videos that show how to apply make-up, depending on the look you hope to achieve. With all that information so readily available, rather than give you each step in detail, I'll give you a summary of some important things to remember, as well as lesser known facts. Most of this will refer to going from male to female, because going from female to male depends on using little or no make-up.

Steps for Female to Male Make-Up Transformation:

Stubble and five o'clock shadow

Adding facial hair

Steps for Male to Female Make-Up Transformation:

Shave. Shave as close as possible at home with a multi-track razor. Even better, visit a barber shop and get a straight edge shave. You'll be smooth as a baby's bottom.

Beard Cover. If you have a dark beard, the skin under your beard will have a bluish tinge from the beard stubble. You can neutralize that blue color with a reddish-tinged cover-up cream. Some specific products are Joe Blasco Blue Neutralizer or Ben Nye Five O'Sharp. Each comes in a range of tones. You can also use a lipstick

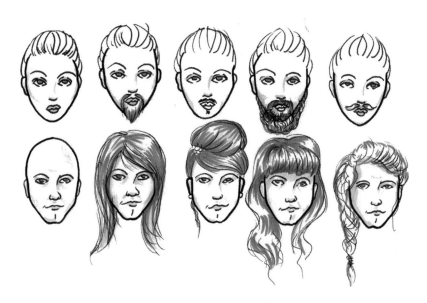

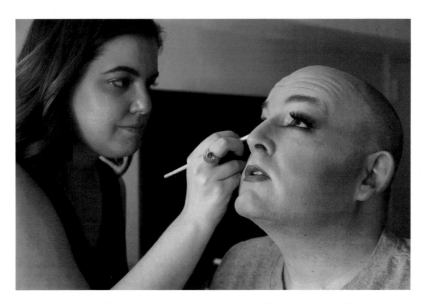

Miss Bridie, dean of make-up, does Bianca. Photo by Daphne Chan.

that is a red or orange tint. Whatever you choose, be sure to apply with a cosmetic sponge and only over the area of your beard. Apply in a rolling motion so that you work the product between each hair follicle.

Foundation. Creams give better coverage than liquids. Choose a cream that matches your skin tone. Don't drag the foundation over the beard cover. Pat on with a sponge, so that you are putting this layer over your beard cover, not mixing the two together.

Powder. Apply loose powder or pressed powder. This step sets your foundation. Anytime you put a dry product over a wet product, it helps set the wet product. It's your choice whether to apply with a brush or a powder puff.

Remember, all your make-up should be applied with upward strokes. Don't drag your face down.

Now you have your canvas and can begin sculpting with high-lights and contours. Contours are powders that are darker than your foundation. Highlights are lighter than your foundation. You will use a contour on any area that you would like to recede and a highlight on any area that you would like to enhance. For instance, narrow your nose by putting a contour down each side and a highlight down the middle.

Male facial structure that is generally different from female: Men have broader jaws and protruding brow bones. Use contour on these areas to downplay them. Highlight nearby areas that you would like to play up.

BIG EYES, BIG LIPS, BIG HAIR

Eyebrows frame your face. If you think they are too bushy or too straggly, it's better to tame them than eliminate them. Unruly brows can be waxed by professionals and/or tweezed and shaped. I don't advise waxing your own, but you can certainly learn to tweeze. Brow stencil kits are a fun way to experiment in re-shaping your brows. Even if you've been tweezing your brows for years, these stencils can give you additional ideas. You can use a soft brow pencil or, for better control, brow powder and a brush to enhance the desired shape. Eyebrows add femininity as well as drama and glamour... all good things.

False eyelashes are a challenge to attach, but well worth the effort. Lashes can be attached as one long strip or individually. In any case, once you have applied eyelash adhesive to the strip or single lash, give the glue a few seconds to dry and get a bit tacky before placement.

Different style lashes create different effects. Thick lashes are more seductive. Lashes where the individual hairs are spread further apart are a more wide awake, alert look. This style can also make you look younger. If the eyelash strip appears to be longer than you need, just snip off a portion from the end. Often strip lashes are graduated. Place the end with the shorter lashes near your nose. If you need to shorten the strip, snip from the longer lashes at the far end of the strip.

Our dean of cosmetology Miss Bridie always uses individual lashes when she does a bride's make-up. If there's a chance tears might flow and lash glue loosen, she'd rather the bride have a single lash fall to her cheek than a whole strip.

As for lashes that last a whole week, choose your practitioner carefully. The glue comes in different grades. If a practitioner uses a cheap product, you may lose a few of your own precious natural lashes when it comes time to remove the false ones. Unfortunately, I speak from experience. Lashes will grow back eventually, but better to keep them safe.

There are plenty of lash enhancement products on the market. Reviews regarding their effectiveness and chance of irritation are mixed. Read those reviews, get personal recommendations. It's best to purchase a product that offers your money back if you are not satisfied. Of course, stop using the product at the first sign of a problem.

Eye liner and eye shadows can enhance the look you are trying to create. They always follow the same rules of art as your foundations. What is dark recedes, what is bright stands out.

The most popular way to apply eye shadow uses three different shades or colors: light, medium and dark. The lightest shade goes across the entire lid. The darkest shade goes in the outer corner of each lid. The medium shade goes above the lid, but not directly under the brow. The area just under the brow is where you will once again use the lightest shade.

Blush is used to highlight your cheekbones or some other area of your face, as well as to give your face a warm, healthy glow. Where you will place your blush depends on the shape of your face and the effect you want to achieve. The classic application is on top of your cheekbone.

As you can see, there can be many steps involved when using make-up to go from male to female. If you feel confident to do these steps on your own, then give yourself the time you need and luxuriate in the process. If you feel overwhelmed, find a make-up artist to do it for you. Enjoy the pampering, because that too is part of the male to female experience. Then get ready to be surprised when you see how good you look.

Or, you can forget about all of the steps and choose only one item of make-up. Can you guess what that is? Why, lipstick, of course. Stain your lips ruby red and there will be no doubt that you are attempting to get in touch with your inner femme. It will be obvious to all who see you and most of all to you whenever you look in the mirror.

Because make-up is the province of women, the use or non-use of it can leave as deep an impression as the product themselves. A woman in search of her inner man can enjoy the delightful freedom of no make-up. You are no longer trying to please, or cover up flaws, or look younger or seduce. You are naturally confident, just as you are.

TATTOO YOU

One of the very first topics that excited my imagination was the art of tattoo. I attended a tattoo convention and wrote about it for a men's magazine. I befriended tattoo artist extraordinaire Spider Webb and learned more about the art and artists: Lyle Tuttle and the old school artists: Bert Grimm, Sailor Jerry, Bob Shaw, Sailor Sid. A primitive art, for some time tattoos were thought to appeal only to sailors or the inebriated. But tattoos are now worn by many and are the mark of the modern primitive. The late, great erotic writer Marco Vassi was definitely gender fluid. His cross gender self was Margo. To celebrate his female essence he had a vulva tattooed on his belly.

Wear a tiny tattoo as a reminder of your inner outlaw, or wear arms full of colors to align yourself with shamans and magic. Those were the two primary reasons I had Spider Webb tattoo a fleur de lis design on my foot. It has become my personal symbol and that of Miss Vera's Finishing School. There is nothing like the feel of the needle for a tattoo or a body piercing to let feel you are alive, and then be a constant reminder.

FINDING YOUR FASHION STYLE

T HERE IS A REASON why the garment business is a multi-billion dollar industry. We all need clothes. Even if you live at a nudist camp, you need to keep a little something on hand for excursions.

Clothing is a great prop to help you break gender barriers and go from male to female or female to male. So how will you dress your cross gender self? Form can follow function or function can follow form.

The right outfit can inspire you to act in a certain way. Lingerie is a great example. Lingerie is the uniform of sex. No matter how you identify your gender, when you dress in sheer nylon, you know that you have exposed

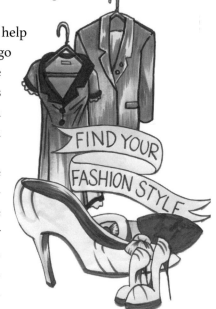

FIND YOUR FASHION STYLE

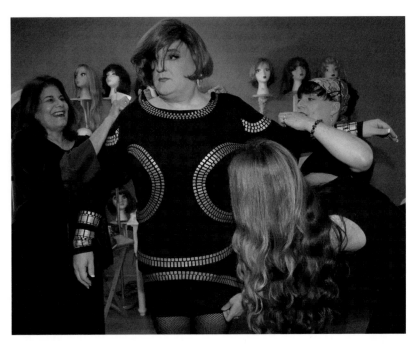

The deans dress Bianca. Photo by Judy Schiller.

yourself; that knowledge is personally exciting and helps you send the message that you are juicy and ready to play.

Function can necessitate form. Maybe you're a woman preparing for a road trip and you want to become more of an expert in car repairs: don that cotton jumpsuit and picture yourself the world's best mechanic. (Of course, often you need to support the look and the wardrobe with practical lessons and decisions to help you accomplish your goals. At Miss Vera's Finishing School, we have an expert faculty and a curriculum of lessons, some of which have to do with presentation, others with skills. In the case of our road warrior, lessons in car repair would be wise. And membership in AAA makes good sense.)

Clothing does exude a kind of magic. Creating a visual image of your cross gender other is a powerful step. My student who initially presented as Patrick stayed up for hours following Patrick's first transformation, staring at the photos we had taken of Patricia.

Those pictures helped Pat to believe life as Patricia was possible and she eventually transitioned.

Today, women have much more freedom with wardrobe, so going from a dress to trousers is not as large a leap as man's going from pants to a skirt. But any change of clothes will have an impact, and the greater the difference in style, the greater the impact on you and

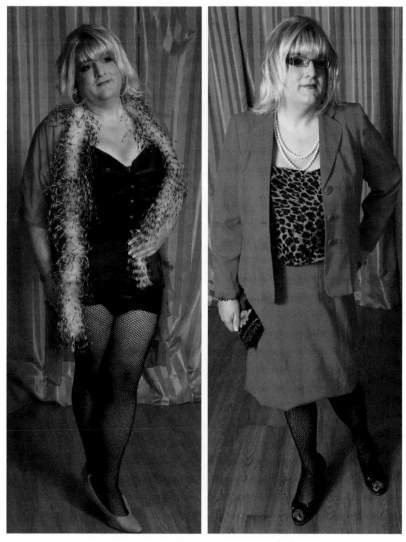

Bianca "night and day." Photo by Judy Schiller.

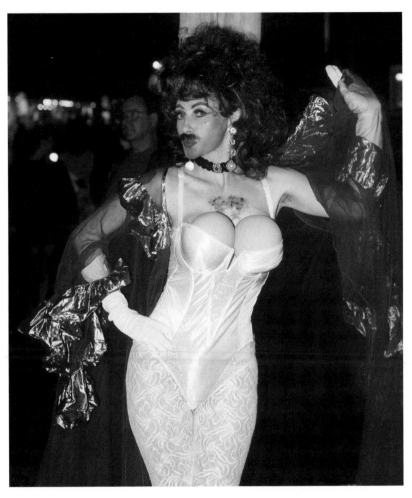

Katharine as drag queen Bubbles Galore. Photo by Annie Sprinkle.

others. Clothing for men originated to provide protection and freedom of movement. In male mode, you will likely cover up more of your body. You may also wear looser garments.

Clothing for women was meant to protect, but also to attract. Women's clothes often follow the shape of the body, and fit closer. A man's jacket that is cut closer to the body, such as an Italian-cut suit, is a more feminine look than a double-breasted blazer. Among the classic looks for men are the business suit, the black leather jacket, the man in uniform, the blue collar – and each of those items has some subcategories.

Some men's looks:

Who wears a business suit? An executive. A dandy.

Who wears a leather jacket? An outlaw (biker or otherwise).

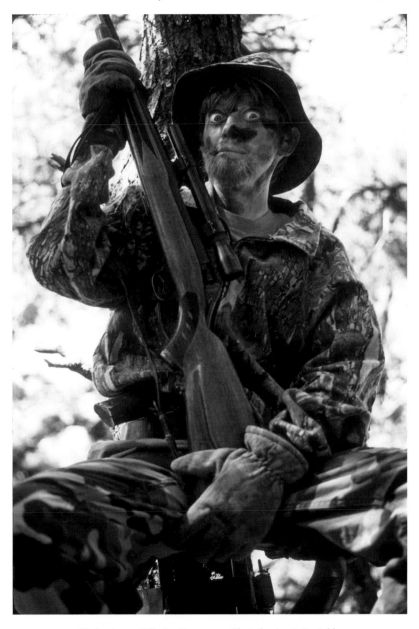

Katharine as Billy Joe Freeman 2. Photo by Annie Sprinkle.

Who wears a uniform? Military, police officers, firemen.
Who wears a blue collar? Mechanics, tradesmen.

Classic looks for women include:
The femme fatale: A clingy sheath that hugs every curve.
Sophisticated career woman: Business suit with skirt.
'50s full skirt: Think Grace Kelly in *Rear Window*.
Fashionista: Designer labels.

Those are just a few of the many, many options. We didn't even touch on the specialty categories such as kinky PVC, latex or leather from the world of BDSM, colorful hippie chic, traditional ethnic, fantasy wardrobe. All of these suggests different qualities: the powerful invulnerability of a skin-tight cat suit, the carefree freedom of fluttery tie-dye, the gracious kimono-clad geisha, the French maid in high heels and ruffles.

Costume play, or "cosplay," is more popular than ever, with a strong influence from Japanese anime and cartoons or manga. This has greatly expanded the range of costumes. Cross gender play is very common in cosplay. You can emulate a character that exists and use this as your role model, or take inspiration from the huge range of costumes and colors to form a new icon uniquely your own. Let your imagination fly.

But suppose you want to keep this simple and choose only one fashion item to announce your cross-gender self. Today, women make that one fashion statement with a fedora. A fedora is a hat with a brim and a crease down the center of the crown. If a fedora isn't your style, try a top hat, a beret, fisherman's cap, baseball cap (visor in front or in back), a Stetson – there are plenty of styles from which to choose, depending on what looks good and sends the message you wish to convey. A hat is a crown, and to wear one takes some confidence. To wear one connotes you have the confidence to carry it off.

For years, the most significant gender-bending item for men was an earring. Emerging these days as a new statement for men is the

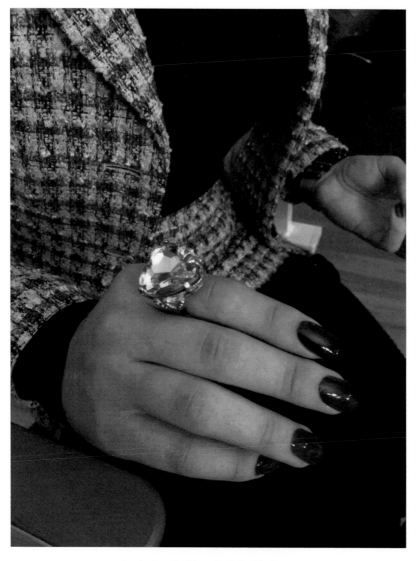

Jessica's nails. Photo by Julia Bingham.

manicure and/or pedicure. In the history-making televised inter-view of Bruce Jenner by Diane Sawyer, Jenner stated that what he most looked forward to post-transition was to wear nail polish long enough for it to chip.

After Caitllin Jenner made her glamorous debut on the cover of *Vanity Fair*, this line about nail polish was cited as proof that Jenner's understanding of womanhood was superficial and limited to the outer trappings. The critics did not understand that nail polish was only a metaphor. The important part of Jenner's statement was not the nail polish, but the chip. Wearing polish long enough to chip meant not having to quickly remove it in order to get back to life as a man, either because you had to present as such for a TV show, or because you had to hide. Chipped polish meant freedom.

Even before I met my husband Stu, he treated himself to a week-ly manicure, and not the clear polish variety. He usually went for deep red nails, and he kept them long. Stu loved to watch people do double-takes when, in the course of everyday situations, they caught a glimpse of his bright talons. Either they said nothing or showered him with compliments.

Manicures also have healing properties. Students have come to my Academy with nails bitten down to the quick. The more they balance their energies by exploring their feminine aspects, the lon-ger their nails grow, and the longer their nails grow, the more calm and confident they become.

HUSBAND/WIFE
SWITCHING

FORM CAN FOLLOW FUNCTION. Or function can follow form.

A married couple, husband and wife, visited my academy for a cross gender exploration. He wasn't a cross-dresser, they had just come for the adventure. They arrived in very casual clothes: he wore a tee-shirt, jeans and a hoodie, she wore jeans, a knit top and sweater.

The couple began by telling me they had trouble communicating. "He just doesn't listen," said the wife. "She's controlling," said the husband.

They'd been together for twelve years, married for ten. This was her second marriage and his first. The couple was in their early forties. From the additional information they gave me, I learned he worked in the building trades and brought home the main paycheck. She took care of their home, and was in charge of their budget. She also earned some money as a housewares rep.

His construction job, which he said he loved, took place on skyscrapers – it was dangerous work. I wondered how steady he would be on four-inch heels. The description of the wife's household management skills made me want to help her get in touch with her inner CEO.

Our starting point was the physical transformation. Two deans led the husband away to change out of his male clothes into feminine lingerie, while two other deans set about giving the wife a more flat-chested appearance by wrapping an ACE bandage around her full bosom. I had picked out a navy blue blazer and trousers for her, but she chose an outfit she thought her husband might actually wear, a black leather jacket and jeans. She wanted to act like him to show him how difficult he could be. The name she chose was Ralph, a salute to Ralph Kramden of *The Honeymooners:* a blue-collar guy, just like her husband.

Suddenly, the husband burst from the dressing room and danced around on tippy-toes, wearing only the gaff – a tight thong to hold down the penis – and a pair of frilly panties. He was a daredevil at work, and apparently an exhibitionist at the academy. Everyone laughed at his performance – everyone except his wife. I realized he had interrupted my discussion with her, claimed all our attention with his antics, and made it difficult for her to be heard.

We transformed the husband and gave his cross gender self the name "Sheila." Sheila wore a form-fitting animal print dress and a blonde wig and pumps, which Sheila handled pretty well for a first-time girl. We always take lots of souvenir photos for our students, but Sheila began taking selfies. This husband was in love with himself as a female.

Meanwhile the wife, "Ralph," had no trouble stomping through a walking class. Ralph impatiently tapped a foot while waiting for

Sheila to finish getting ready, a scenario they'd played out many times in reverse.

Sheila was unstoppable and seemingly out of control – but was that really the case? Was the husband just having fun, making jokes and being foolish, or were we witnessing how this couple normally communicated?

The wife had said, "He doesn't listen." The husband had said, "She's too controlling." By seeming to go out of control, he was taking charge.

The husband's behavior dominated his wife. The couple were about the same size; he was a bit taller and more slim, she rounder. But now, the wife seemed to be shrinking as her husband acted out.

I decided to go back to my original thought for the wife, which was to dress her in executive clothes and support her inner CEO. I reasoned she would then be less familiar to her husband. He was a union guy and used to hanging out with the other workers, not dealing with management – so we'd turn her into management.

In these new more upscale and stylish duds, the wife in male role fell immediately into a swagger. She was now cock of the walk. A new name was chosen: Ralph became Raymond. The name just came to her; it means protector or "king of the world." The wife liked that.

Raymond, as opposed to sloppy Ralph, was someone who was very careful about his appearance. We pulled her long hair back into a tight braid.

A remarkable thing happened. Sheila, the husband, began flirting with Raymond, the wife. Sheila fluttered her eyelashes and flipped her hair. Raymond patted his thigh, inviting Sheila, her feminine husband, to take a seat. Sheila sat, and compared to Raymond's more ample chest, seemed much smaller.

They looked at each other eye to eye. They moved their faces closer. Raymond took Sheila's face in her hands. Sheila pulled back and wisecracked, "Don't mess my lipstick." Raymond sighed, frustrated with her husband's constant jokes. But then Sheila said, "You know, ever since I was in high school, I've felt insecure about my

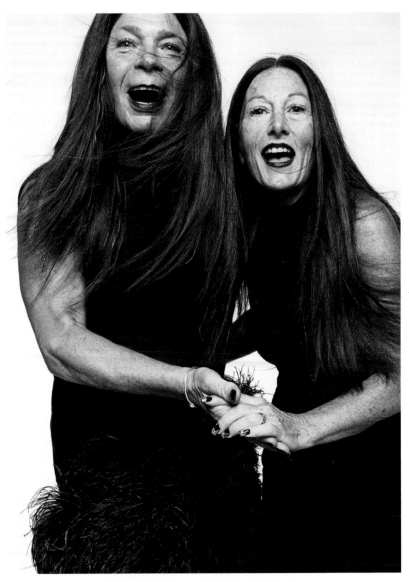

Amy & Trish. Photo by Philippe Vogelenzang.

size, but as a girl... I'm just right." Raymond beamed at her man in a dress. She took his made up face in her hands and asked, "Who's your Daddy? Sheila, who's the boss now?"

"You are," said Sheila, as they shared a long kiss.

Finding the right clothes, the right look for this couple helped them to step outside of themselves and relate in a different way. They made a new connection.

"Spread your legs," I told Raymond. Then I helped Sheila to the floor to kneel between Raymond's legs. Now Sheila was in the position he'd always urged his wife to occupy, while Raymond, the masculinized wife, sat above, gazing down at her feminized husband. We'd created a bulge in Raymond's pants, so she had a nice package, but it was made out of cloth, so not really to be put to practical use. But the couple seemed ready to play, so I handed Raymond a dildo, which she placed within easy reach of Sheila's mouth.

"Go ahead, show me how it's done," said Raymond. "You always tell me that I could do better, so show me how you like it. Be my sweet cocksucker. Inspire me."

Sheila rose to the challenge. The husband put his mouth around Raymond's wide shaft and swallowed down deep, then came back up slowly.

"You're so good, I think I'll hire you out," said Raymond.

"Why should today be different?" said Sheila. "You pimp me out almost every day. Monday through Friday, I work for you."

This small act of role play brought up the two topics most affected by life in the gender binary – topics which you, whether single or partnered, must address to get the most benefit from your cross gender explorations. These are sex and money.

Whether you are single or partnered, awareness of your relationships to sex and money is essential. In the case of this couple, they'd lost the sense of partnership they had enjoyed in the beginning of their marriage. They were still a couple, but each felt very much alone, and acted as such. Each felt unappreciated by the other.

They'd fallen into patterns of withholding. The wife withheld sex; the husband withheld respect. But what they wanted from each other, they had to first give to themselves. The costumes helped, as did a third pair of eyes, mine, to view their interactions.

The wife needed to believe in her own expertise as a money manager and communicate that expertise to her husband. The husband needed to acknowledge the joy he took in his job for its own sake, not as a way to escape from responsibilities of the house.

A visit to an accountant helped the couple to see that they were really on solid footing financially, thanks to both their efforts. The wife learned she could loosen the purse strings and plan for the fun vacation her husband wanted. The husband learned what a good job the wife had done, not only with the money he brought into the house, but with the additional money she earned in her own burgeoning business. They hired a housekeeper one day a week so the wife could spend more time nurturing that business.

The wife felt empowered, the husband felt relief. She no longer played the role of the frustrated housewife. He no longer played the role of the downtrodden spouse. Released from the confines of outmoded gender binary thinking, each felt more whole, more supported by the other, more fortunate, and, happily, more sexy.

WORK THAT BODY:
MOVEMENT
AND VOICE

WORK THAT BODY: MOVEMENT AND VOICE

I'VE WATCHED MANY STUDENTS as they follow the instructions of Miss Julia, our dean of high heels, and attempt to walk in a more feminine manner. While their legs move, it's really the upper body, their shoulders, that they accentuate. I feel as if I am watching some ancient strut in which the male presents the widest part of his body to say, "Look at me. See how big and strong I am." They stand with their feet planted firm on the floor and spread a shoulder-width apart. Men take control of the earth. They walk, they stand and they sit with legs spread, leaving plenty of room for their genitals, the source of their manhood, to rest comfortably.

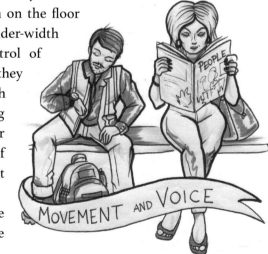

Men don't move their hips – shaking the

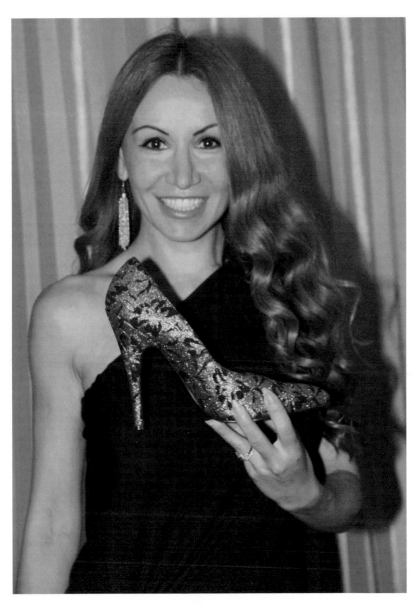

Miss Julia, dean of high heels. Photo by Judy Schiller.

buttocks is what women do to attract a mate. For Eros, attracting a mate, perpetuating the species, is women's work. Going from female to male, you will wear wide flat shoes. You will sit with legs apart.

You will take up more space. Going from male to female, lessons in high heels will raise your buttocks to provocative heights.

No matter which way you are crossing the gender border, good posture is essential. Some men think that to slouch will make them look smaller and hence more feminine, or a woman might slouch to look more like a cave man. But slouching can have a negative effect on the psyche, and I prefer to keep you upright and upbeat.

YOUR VOICE

Trans men have an easier time changing the pitch of their voice, because a lower pitch is a benefit when they take additional testosterone. Trans women can find that changing the pitch of their voice is more of a challenge. Our Dean of Voice, Miss Judy, does not teach our male students to speak in falsetto. It not only sounds artificial, it puts a strain on the vocal cords. We teach our male to female students to elongate vowels and enunciate the plosive sounds, d, p, t, to give a more refined speech. Most important, in going from male to female, we teach our student to put more emotion into their female vocabulary, use more adjectives and be more descriptive. Women use more of a storytelling form. Men make statements.

For the purpose of finding your cross-gender icon, I think it's more to speak up, to not be afraid to express yourself and to communicate honestly. To accomplish that, it's more important to focus – not on the voice that comes out of your mouth– but the voice in your head, your inner voice.

If you spend some time listening to your thoughts, you may be surprised to find that a large percentage of the things you say to yourself are negative. The purpose of creating a cross gender icon is to enhance your options and abilities, to do things that you did not think were possible for you before, to grow. You may have spent an entire lifetime believing these were things you cannot do. Now, it's time to silence that negative thinking by re-training that inner voice with affirmations and positivity.

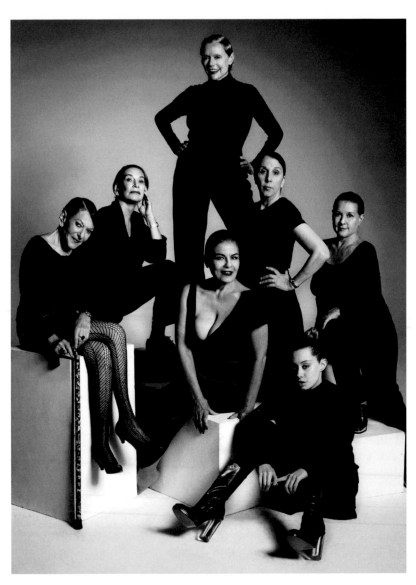

Miss Vera's Finishing School Faculty (clockwise, l to r). Topaz Lennard, Mariette Pathy Allen, Maryanne Byington, Judy Pollak, Deborah Raposa, Amanda Flowers, Veronica Vera. Photo by Philippe Vogelenzang.

Cross Gender Fun for All

Let's start with a basic thought: your ability to create your cross gender self. First, listen to your current thoughts:

- "I'm too much of a guy/gal to ever make this work."
- "I'll end up looking foolish."
- "I don't have the right clothes."
- "I'm too big/small."
- "This is too much work."

Now let's spin those thoughts to positive affirmations.

- "There are many ways to access my cross gender self. I'm sure I can find a way that works for me."
- "I'm excited to look different."
- "I don't need an entire new wardrobe, the smallest change can make a big difference."
- "My actual size matters less than the image that I project."
- "Every step in this process is fun and illuminating."

You can also use this affirming process to change your thinking about more specific details of your cross gender exploration. For instance, your sex appeal.

LEARNING NEW SKILLS

As many options as you have to change your appearance, so there are options to change your behavior as you explore this new identity. You might want to take a some lessons in cooking or carpentry to support your cross gender self. You can find a YouTube.com video about nearly any subject. Three fundamental areas that I will discuss here are your sex life, money matters and your relationships with others.

It's really true that practice makes perfect, so don't expect to change overnight, or simply from reading this book. My goal is to raise your awareness of options, to prepare you with more information. These three topics – sex, money, how we relate to others

– have something in common: the way you function in these areas has to a great extent been learned, usually handed down to you by your parents.

But you are not your parents, nor are you restricted by the confines of a gender binary way past its prime. So if you feel some lack in your sex life, your financial dealings, or the way you relate to others, be aware you have the freedom, even a responsibility, to change.

Nothing happens in a vacuum. In the United States it is now possible for two people of any gender to marry. That means that – except for giving birth – the role of mother, that has always been fulfilled by a female, along with a list of attributes ascribed to woman, may now be fulfilled by a man. The same goes for the role of father, which can be fulfilled by a woman. Parents are now two humans of any gender. Parenting can also be accomplished by one person in both roles.

The best way to give to yourself and to contribute to future generations, is to discover more and more of the options available to you for your own growth and pleasure that may then be passed down to others. This is how we have arrived at the current level of understanding.

PRACTICAL LESSONS

Once you have identified the qualities and talents that you would like your icon to possess, we need to give you practical steps or lessons to support you. At Miss Vera's Finishing School, this is where the deans come in – with practical lessons in voice, movement, make-up skills, comfort with being out and about, as well as sharing with a partner and others. And, most of all, self-acceptance.

But if you would like your icon to help you with learning to build a business, cook dinner, repair a leaky faucet, be a more adventurous lover... then we need to find ways to facilitate that part of your education. This is where the lessons that I described regarding voice class are especially helpful. It's likely that for years, you have spent many hours telling yourself you are not good at these talents and qualities that you want your icon to possess. Time to write your affirmations and play the tapes of your inner voice, the one that has confidence in your abilities.

Now reach out for the help you need. Either find a teacher or class that will help you learn to do something yourself, or find an expert who can do the job so that you can move on to something else.

GONE ARE THE DAYS when sex information was hard to find, grossly inaccurate, or overly academic. Sex information is everywhere, and much of it is dispensed by passionate experts in clear and cheerful style. In fact, there so much information you may feel a bit overwhelmed. So let's get down to the basics.

By now, you know that my entire career was influenced by a desire to find my own answers, discover my personal sexual truth. Here is what I believe. After doing much practical research in the field of human sexuality, I coined a statement that I call my Theory of Sexual Evolution: "We all have personal sexual needs, desires, experiences, feelings and attitudes that have formed over time. Some of this was present at birth, much more followed as we grew. Bottom line: *You have the right to be who you are as sexual human being, as long as you respect the rights of others.*"

Procreation is essential for survival, but no less important is sexual pleasure. Your sexual energy contributes to your good health and creativity.

In 1989, at the request of my friend Annie Sprinkle, I authored a document to coincide with her performance, *Post Porn Modernist*. The Post Porn Modernist Manifesto I wrote was signed by Candida Royalle, Betty Dodson, Frank and Debbie Moore and Annie herself, as well as many other artistic and sexual pioneers. It read:

"We of the Post Porn Modernist Movement
Embrace our genitals as part, not separate from our spirits.
We utilize sexually explicit words, pictures, performances to communicate our ideas and emotions.
We denounce sexual censorship as anti-art and inhuman.
We empower ourselves by this attitude of sex-positivism.
And with this love of our sexual selves we have fun, heal the world and endure."

Guilty or not guilty? Have you ever felt guilty about sex? One reason to feel guilt about sex is if you break the trust of a partner or help another person to break their trust. But do you ever feel guilty about your secret dreams? Or about actions that involve only yourself? Why is that?

Guilt can be an aphrodisiac. To do something you consider forbidden can make it all the more exciting. Guilt can also be a way to express love. You've done something that, as a child, your parents told you was wrong, so you feel guilty. You suffer guilt in order to prove your love for your parents. Guilt can help maintain your sense of security. You know there are rules – and, even though your dreams are forbidden, the fact that you know you are wrong means that you can still belong to the same community.

Do you see the fallacies behind this thinking? If I simply said to you, "Guilt and love are the same thing," I have no doubt you would argue with me. If I said, "Guilt and security are the same," you would differ. "Guilt and pleasure are equal"? I don't think so. Love, security, pleasure are rich and fulfilling. Guilt is tiny and cheap. To accept guilt as a replacement for love, security or pleasure is to short-change yourself. It takes more courage to acquire

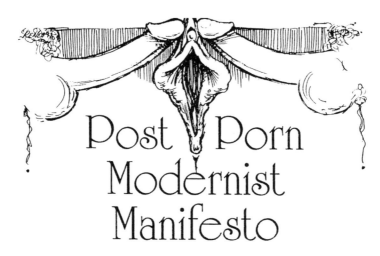

Post Porn Modernist Manifesto

LET IT BE KNOWN to all who read these words or witness these events that a new awareness has come over the land. We of the POST PORN MODERNIST MOVEMENT face the challenge of the Rubber Age by acknowledging this moment in our personal sexual evolutions and in the sexual evolution of the planet.

Post Porn Modernists celebrate sex as the nourishing, life-giving force.

We embrace our genitals as part, not separate, from our spirits.

We utilize sexually explicit words, pictures and performances to communicate our ideas and emotions.

We denounce sexual censorship as anti-art and inhuman.

We empower ourselves by this attitude of sex-positivism.

And with this love of our sexual selves we have fun, heal the world and endure.

–Vera, June 1989

Your name (if you dare): _____

Post Porn Modernist Manifesto. Drawing by Rene "IATBA" Moncada.

self-knowledge, but the effort is exciting and the rewards are real and well worth it.

Cross-gender play can be the perfect catalyst in liberating your erotic life. Up until now, your sexual practice may have been limited by your identity as a man or a woman. For decades, even centuries, sexual experience was considered a favorable quality in a man, while a woman lost value once she was deflowered. Thankfully, that kind of thinking is outmoded, but some remnants may still be embedded in your psyche.

Are you a man who would like to be pursued rather than always feeling you are the one in pursuit? Or, though you are a man, perhaps you feel inhibited and desire to know your inner wild woman. Are you a woman who is always "the good girl," yet yearns to be a playboy? And what if you are sexually attracted to someone of the same gender? How does your understanding of gender mesh with your sexual orientation?

The human body is equipped with enough holes and appendages for you to give and experience pleasure, whether you are alone or with anyone of any gender. In addition to what your physical body provides, there is the erogenous zone of the mind, plus a billion-dollar industry of toys and electronics to help you. Your options are seemingly endless.

You may think that your choice of sexual partners remains constant, but that is not necessarily so. First, sexual energy is very powerful. You can be turned on by watching others who are turned on: that is the power of pornography. Whether you act on your feelings is another matter.

Just yesterday, I had lunch with my student Brad, who enjoys cross-dressing. Brad is very happily married – in fact, Brad's wife encouraged him to come to the Academy to reveal his anima. We transformed the student and discovered his anima, Barbara. Now, that she was unleashed, Brad confided that he dreamed his femmeself Barbara could give oral pleasure to a man. The student asked "I have two questions: 1) Do you think that I really want to do that? 2) Do you think I ever will do that?" Brad said he felt guilty having these fantasies. I told Brad: We cannot police our fantasies.

Brad had been sharing his Academy experiences with his wife. He created a Facebook page for Barbara, and Barbara received numerous proposals for trips, encounters, and quite a few penis photos from male admirers. Brad had shared all of this correspondence with his wife. They'd had quite a few chuckles about some of the more outlandish offers. But Brad had not shared with his wife the fantasy that Barbara would orally pleasure a man. Brad said that this particular fantasy frightened him.

In answer to Brad's two questions I said, 1) Yes, I think you would like to live that fantasy, and 2) I don't believe you will actually do it... right now. I told him his actions were in his control, but because he had done something out of character, namely not shared this desire with his wife, he felt guilty and not in control. He just didn't feel like himself – and he wasn't, he was Barbara.

However, if he could accept Barbara as part of Brad, all one wonderfully complex human being, then he would feel empowered. He could share his feelings with his wife, though sharing might temporarily defuse the excitement of his guilty secret. But together they could decide a next step. Perhaps she would agree he could explore that fantasy; perhaps she would explore it with him. I told Brad there was a third question he might ask me: 3) Given a different situation, namely that his wife knew of his desires, would he ever fulfill that fantasy? Then the answer could be "Yes."

A lot of people come to me to be a guide, but if you are in a committed relationship, you may have the very best guide and the very best playmate in your partner. You'll never know if you don't ask.

Marriage then, marriage now. The purpose of marriage is for two people to join together and support each other in creating a home and family, as they define home and family. Think about the most commonly accepted words in the wedding ceremony question: "Do you _____ take _____ to be your lawfully wedded spouse, to love and to cherish, for richer for poorer, in sickness and in health, from this day forward for as long as you both shall live"? It is a union of two people.

Sometimes the words "forsaking all others" are added. This question dates back centuries, to a time when there were many assumptions about marriage. Marriage was between one man and one woman; the man was the head of the house; at one time the woman was thought to be the man's chattel. Monogamy and fidelity were assumed to mean the same thing. But are they? Do they need to be? If you are married, or thinking of getting married, it is up to you and your spouse to answer that question.

Polyamory. Happily, more and more people are discovering the benefits of polyamory, the practice of being in a committed and loving relationship with more than one person, not all of whom are necessarily having sex with one another. I have long recommended polyamory as an option to couples who consult my academy. Polyamory is a wonderful choice for committed couples who value honesty and trust, but are attracted to sex with other partners. It's particularly helpful when one or both partners is trans or bisexual. You can be single and be polyamorous too.

"Polyamory" refers to romantic love with more than one person, honestly, ethically, and with the full knowledge and consent of all concerned. Polyamory often involves multiple long-term committed relationships, either separately or together, but it can also come in many different forms. Some examples are:

- Open polyamory (committed open relationship or open marriage), in which the partners involved remain open to the possibility of additional loves and relationships;
- Polyfidelity, in which three or more people commit to having a closed relationship with each other and not getting involved with anyone outside the group;
- Single polyamorists, who may have several loves without a primary commitment to any one person, and who may or may not be looking for long-term partnership.

Role Play. Create a solo portrait or engage with a partner. With you and a partner in cross gender modes, role play naturally follows. It can be guided. You can assume roles of sheer fantasy or assume a more practical bent. Choose from the classics: teacher and student, client and whore, pirate and wench, secretary and boss. When you engage with a partner there is likely to be an exchange of power: one of you is in charge, the other follows. This power exchange may be just the opposite of what usually happens in your sexual and/or non-sexual relations. Not all fantasies are meant to be realized. You can dress the part but not act the part, just get in touch with your dreams. Your everyday self can be faithful and monogamous, but you can imagine a cross gender self who loves to play the field and make conquests. Allowing yourself the freedom to acknowledge your desires makes for self-acceptance and empowerment.

Dominance and submission. The sexual practice most obviously involved in power exchange is BDSM, bondage, discipline and sado-masochism. All have their bases in dominance and submission. Tops and bottoms. The top runs the sex, the bottom follows. This is the realm of kinky sex.

The word "kink" is particularly appropriate. A kink is defined as a curve that goes back on itself, and kinky sex is often associated with our early erotic experiences, many of which stem from childhood. An exploration of these realms can teach you a lot.

Exploring dominance and submission was very liberating for me in that it was a relief from the repression imposed by my parents, their religion and 1950s thinking. Dominant/submissive role play can give you permission to do what you've always wanted to do but needed some support to try.

The summer that I spent with Jeanette Luther, aka Ms. Antoinette, who became my mentor and one of my dearest friends, helped me to own my sexual self. I wore catsuits and ultra-sexy gear, and went back and forth between dominance and submission, going from femme to femme fatale. I didn't cross gender borders, but my partner did. Perhaps if I had, I might have enjoyed the benefits of wearing a strap-on many years sooner.

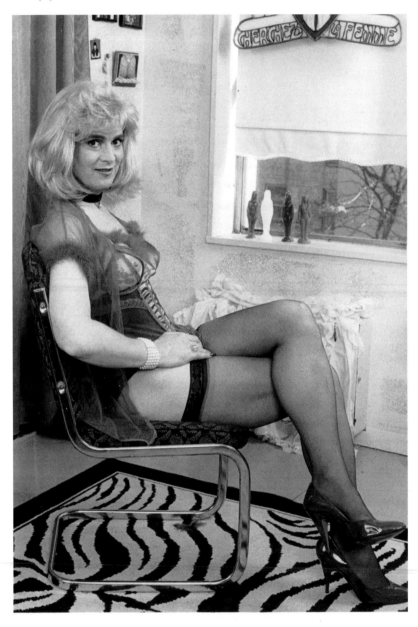

Sexy Michelle. Photo by Barbara Nitke.

Once I left the special experience of Ms. Antoinette, I continued these explorations for some time. To me, this was sex as theater and a very artistic process. When that experience no longer fit, when I wanted a different kind of intimacy, I moved on.

The main purpose in creating your cross gender self is to increase your options, to grow. Awareness is a partner in that growth.

Virgin/sexual experience. The character in the movie *40 Year Old Virgin* was not news to me. I know plenty of you exist, just as there are plenty of you who long to feel like a virgin, again and again. To be a virgin can be your choice, but if you are and prefer to be otherwise, you have many resources. Across the country, there are sexuality boutiques and sex-positive therapists who can help virgins not only learn more from books but have practical experience.

My good friends Tamar and Raymond Reilly are sex surrogates with advanced degrees in human sexuality and a code of ethics required by this profession. They work through recommendations from therapists to bring more people to pleasure.

What if you prefer to leave your former sex life behind and start fresh? It can be an interesting experiment to identify your cross gender icon as a virgin or even celibate: put sex out of your mind for a time and see what or who begins to take up that space. Enjoy the access your cross gender self may provide to be open to a more expanded sexual orientation. We all have bodies equipped with enough erotic avenues to experience pleasure with anyone of any gender. Just being open to the thought can open your heart more to others and to yourself, heighten your sense of security, lessen stress and thus improve your health.

Penetrating observation. Let's talk about the most common shift in sexual positions when you explore your cross gender other. The penis endowed male is the penetrator, the vagina endowed female, the receiver. If you have not yet experienced the opposite, your cross gender self offers that liberty.

For all of my life, I have experienced the pleasure and the inflow of energy that accompanies vaginal penetration. It helped me to understand why many of the students who visited my academy dreamed of being the ones in that position.

"*Penetration feels lovely. It feels so good to be opened, to be filled, to be at the receiving end of a long, slow thrust of passion, or short quick ones, for that matter. When you are penetrated, the body is like a furnace that is stoked, and the heat which is your sexual energy starts to rise, carried on your breath to other parts of your body. The rising of energy is always part of the sexual process, but penetration starts that process in the most swift and sure way.*" So I wrote in the sex education chapter of my first book, *Miss Vera's Finishing School for Boys Who Want to Be Girls*.

I am now happy to report new insights from the perspective of my cross gender self.

It is only very recently that I have become proficient in the use of a strap-on. Providence, or maybe my angel Stu, sent me a new lover for continued research.

Over the years, try as I might, I always felt awkward with a dildo, either holding it or wearing, but practice makes perfect. I now know how the other half lives and I like it.

I chose a two-legged harness for ease of maneuverability. My male-to-female lover and I had tried a number of positions in which I stood while my girl bent over the bed, or got down on all fours while I knelt on the bed behind her.

These positions had some bene-fits: my lover greatly enjoyed the experience of being penetrated, but neither position felt all that exciting to me. I didn't feel that we were really connect-ed. We decided to go for reverse missionary, me on top, my lover on bot-tom, face to face. It took a few tries before I had the strap-on in the right posi-tion, but then I did. My girl's strong arms and legs wrapped around me. My lover was holding on for dear life. I plunged deep and reached the depths of his need. I thought, "This must be what it's like for guys. No wonder men feel so powerful fucking women when they can feel this explosive hunger in response to their cocks!" It was the first time that I realized the hugely beneficial energy of being a cocksman. Bravo, Señor.

Sexual energy. By now it's likely you've noticed that when I discuss sex, I refer to energy. The practice of sex is the way we activate energy, share energy and merge energy. If you think of sex simply as a physical act centered in the body, you are short-changing yourself.

When you engage in sexual activity, either with yourself or with others, you contribute your energy to the universal life force, a force that is gender neutral, gender fluid. In metaphysical thought, we have not only a physical body but an astral body, a mental body, a spiritual body – and, through these bodies of energy, we connect to every living thing and to all creation. You may identify as a particular gender, but your existence is bigger and more free.

My friends Annie Sprinkle and Elizabeth Stephens have popularized the philosophy called "ecosex." Their motto is "Earth as lover, not Earth as mother"; they are married, not only to each other, but together they have married the sea and the stars, the snow, the dirt, all parts of the earth, in order to demonstrate that we all share the same life force. We are all one. Expand your awareness and your sexual options can kiss the sky.

Other disciplines that focus on sex as an energetic practice emphasize the spiritual aspects of sex. Western religions most often repress sex, but Eastern religions and philosophies include sex as essential to life. Western religions focus on sex as physical acts to create new life. Eastern philosophies see the purpose of sex as energy, to sustain and enhance everyday existence.

The most popular examples of these Eastern philosophies are Tantra and Taoism. Tantra, as taught in the U.S., is a westernized version of an Asian practice which influenced both Hinduism and

Buddhism. In Tantra, sexual energy is exchanged primarily through the breath.

On a visit to India, I was eager to view the erotic temples of Khajuraho. The temples were constructed in about 1000 CE by devotees of what we now refer to as Tantra. The walls of these temples are covered with carvings of people engaged in a variety of sexual positions, designed to give pleasure and also to heal. The sex acts facilitate the exchange of breath, which is the artery of pleasure. In the Kama Sutra, known as the Hindu bible of sex, the pursuit of pleasure is an important aim in life on the path of enlightenment.

Taoists revere the human primordial life force, which is referred to as "chi," and chi is part of the primordial life force of the entire universe. In Tantra and the Tao, the purpose of your sexual energy is to contribute to your chi, and your chi contributes to the chi of every living thing. When you use your body with awareness in the service of pleasure, the energy derived from that pleasure is good for you and the entire planet.

Contemplating your life from a new perspective, in this case, that of your cross gender icon, may result in a change in your philosophy, with accompanying wardrobe. Will it be a monk's robe or a sari skirt? Change your clothes and you just may change your mind.

IF WE COULD TALK TO THE ANIMALS

A wonderful exhibit at the Museum of Sex in New York City describes the the sex lives of animals. One of the creatures you can learn about there is a tiny fish named the Blue Banded Gobie. Here is the bio: Blue Banded Gobies live in harems of one male and four to six females. The male is socially dominant and the females live as subordinates. However, when the male is removed, the highest-ranking female assumes a position of dominance. She rapidly begins to express male-typical social and sexual behavior (gender change). Within weeks her gonads, accessory structures (prostate-like glands), external genitalia, endocrine profiles, brain chemistry and growth rate become male (sex

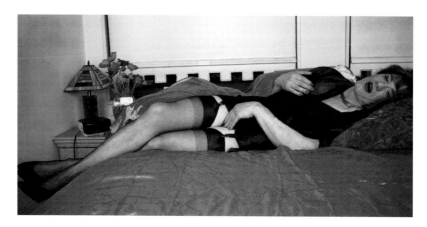
Marsha. Photo by Sophia Wallace.

change). Remarkably, if this newly transformed male is then socially subordinated by a more aggressive male, the transformed male will revert back to female function.

Do you think only females become pregnant? That's not so, if you are a seahorse. In species with sex role reversal, females make eggs faster than males can incubate them. In some species, males spend more time than females tending the young. This is referred to as sex-role reversal.

The most well-known examples of sex-role reversals include seahorses and their relatives, the pipe fish and sea dragons. Male seahorses have pouches on their stomachs, into which the females lay eggs. The males become pregnant and eventually give birth to the young. In pipefish, eggs attach to the undersides of the males, and in some species the eggs are protected by a flap of skin.

In 2015, the United States finally acknowledged the right of same-sex couples to marry, but same-sex relationships are far from rare in nature. Displays of courtship, mounting, sexual stimulation, pair-bonding and parenting behaviors have been documented in over five hundred animal species. With all of this amazing variety happening in nature, how could we who are also a part of nature expect that our sex lives and orientations would be all neat and tidy?

Why spend so much time discussing sex with you? Because the more we accept the complexities of sexuality, the more we can accept and love ourselves and others. Too often guilt inhibits us, or is used as a method of control by others, and there is no area where we are more vulnerable than in our often messy sex lives. We are in the midst of a time of great love and healing – examining the fallacies of the gender binary as you explore your cross gender self is a way to keep the momentum going, for us and for generations to come.

MONEY,
HONEY

MONEY,
HONEY

HOW DO YOU THINK your financial life as been influenced by the gender in which you live? It's natural to make some immediate assumptions – because a fact of the gender binary system is that for centuries, men have earned and currently earn more than women. An important thing to remember is, you are not your bank account.

All those sayings about money have the ring of truth, especially "money can't buy happiness." Many of the students who visit Miss Vera's Academy hold high-salaried positions in their male roles. The money brings them financial stability, but not the happiness that comes from living a more well-balanced life. They look with envy on the lives of the women earning far less than they are, thinking that these women have more time for fun and a different kind of security.

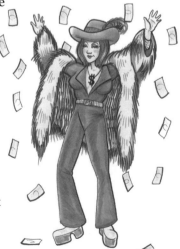

The positions these students hold are confinements, so they come to the Academy to be released from their emotional straitjackets. It's not wearing make-up and a pretty new outfit that does the trick. Dressed in these clothes, they are able to let down their guard and not only allow, but reach for, feelings and emotions that in their more familiar identity seem unattainable or dangerous.

Someone living in the male world fears others may not respect him if he appears in any way sissified. A loss of respect is equated with reduced income. But the security that comes with living an authentic emotional life enhances self-respect, and that is priceless.

And what if your gender is female? Has your conscious or unconscious thinking held you back from having a good relationship with money? I thought facing my sexual issues was a challenge. But that was nothing compared with learning to release a healthy cash flow. Today, young women are encouraged to be financially independent. But many of us grew up expecting financial security as part of the marriage package. Many still do.

Are you in harmony in your relationship with money? If not, this is an area in which your cross gender self can help? If you are a woman, turn your checkbook over to your inner CEO. What grade would he give? If you are a man, compare how much time you spend earning money, to how much time you enjoy the leisure time it can bring. Time is money, after all. Money lost can be regained, but it usually takes time. Time lost is gone.

How healthy is your time/money balance? The status of that balance will influence the relationship you have with family and friends. It will also affect your health.

You may think of money as something tangible, paper and coins that can be measured. But two things to remember: money is fluid and wealth is immeasurable. None of us is meant to hold on to our money forever. Money is meant to pass from hand to hand, stirring energy as it passes. The more you understand about how money works, the more money works for you, not the other way around.

Money is a tool to facilitate creativity, as is time. What do you wish to create? A work of art, a new home, education, ice cream every Saturday? The best things in life are free: a sunset, a bird's song... but even those can be missed if you are not aware of your budget.

YOUR RELATIONSHIPS WITH OTHERS

How will you maintain the benefits you've gained through your cross gender icon? Your support will come from the people with whom you surround yourself. If you've wanted to become more calm and serene, you will need to look at people and situations with a careful eye. Who or what supports you in your endeavors, who or what pushes all your buttons in negative ways? With growth, there is change. If your relationship with someone does not support the change you want in yourself, though you've tried to make it work, you will need to let that relationship go – or at least give it far less of your time. You will fill that time with people and events that do support your goals and add to your options.

There is no age at which we need to stop growing – in fact, just the opposite. By continuing to grow, you discover that fountain of youth.

Cross Gender Fun for All

CONCLUSION

CONCLUSION

MY PURPOSE HAS BEEN to give you a new way of looking at yourself – whether in the mirror or in your mind's eye – to increase your options to be. I hope I've succeeded.

I also hope that you will allow and encourage others to do the same. The world of today has less need for division and more need for union. Be united in your own humanity – your male and your female essence – and you can give birth to a richer, more expanded version of yourself, of your relationships, and of the world.

Nothing less will do.

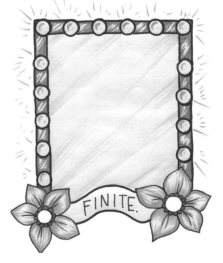

FINITE.

WHAT ARE THE AREAS OF STUDY you might choose to support your cross gender identity and fulfill your goals? Here are some places to start. Some may be perfect for you in your quest. In any case, these suggestions will give you some direction in where to look.

ARTISTS

Diane Torr. Author, *Sex, Drag and Male Roles.* "Man For A Day" is the feature documentary by Katarina Peters that documents Diane Torr's acclaimed workshops. *www.DianeTorr.com.*

Stuart Cottingham aka "Misty Madison." Stu's archive includes the story of Misty in words, photos and videos. *www.StuartCottingham.com.*

Kate Bornstein. Gender Outlaw. *www.katebornstein.com.*

Leon Mostovoy. Photographer and transgender man Leon Mostovoy created The Transfigure Project as a "celebration of bodies the transcend the gender binary." It's a flip book that invites you to mix and match the body parts of nude transgender individuals who bared all for Mostovoy's camera. The online version is an invitation to play and to comment. *www.thetransfigureproject.com*

Annie Sprinkle. All of Annie's art is inspiring. Of particular interest to cross gender explorers are "The Sluts and Goddesses Video WorkShop" and "Linda, Les and Annie, the first Female to Male Love Story," both available from *www.anniesprinkle.org.*

Mariette Pathy Allen. The "Margaret Mead" of transgender studies. Mariette's books of photography and writings based on intimate interviews provide fantastic archive of the transgender phenomenon. Her reseach now takes her around the globe. *www.marietteallen.com.*

Linda Montano. Seminal performance artist whose motto is "Life is Art." Linda is mentor to me, Annie Sprinkle and countless others. *www.lindamontano.com.*

Franklin Furnace. An archive of performance art. Sign up for their "Goings On" newsletter to learn more about who is performing where and what opportunities are offered to support your art life. *www.franklinfurnace.org.*

CARS

Auto Repair for Dummies by Deanna Sclar (2008). Paperback and Kindle.

How Cars Work by Tom Newton. Originally written for teens.

COMMUNITY

Centerlink. This site helps communities form LGBT centers, connects centers with one another, and provides a map which will help you find a center near you. Centers are great places to find information and comrades. *www.lgbtcenters.org.*

TransGender Conferences. Thanks to the Trans Guys for assembling the most information all in one place. Visit the site *transguys. com/ref/2016-trans-conference-guide.*

FASHION

Museum at FIT. Fashion Institute of Technology. Seventh Avenue at 27th Street, NYC, 10001. Valerie Steele, director and chief curator. *www.fitnyc.edu.*

Costume Institute at Metropolitan Museum of Art. 1000 Fifth Avenue @ 82nd Street, NYC, 10028. *www.metmuseum.org.*

FOOD

How to Cook Everything, The Basics: All You Need to Make Great Food by Mark Bittman (2012).

HOME IMPROVEMENT

The Complete Do-it-Yourself Manual, Newly Updated by Editors of Family Handyman (Readers Digest, 2014).

INTELLECTUAL PURSUITS

A Very Short Introduction Series (Oxford University Press). Described as "stimulating ways in to new subjects." Want to know about accounting, the blues, cosmology...Indian philosophy, spirituality... witchcraft? A few hundred different subjects are covered by experts in individual pocket sized guides. If you want to learn more, each book in the series includes a list for further reading. Talk about expanding your mind!

LEGAL

Transgender Legal Defense and Education Fund. This group is committed to ending discrimination based on gender identity and expression. They've got their hands full with public education, test-care litigation, direct legal services and public policy efforts. Name changes and bathrooms are just two tiny parts of this picture. *www.transgenderlegal.org.*

Jamison Green. His firm Jamison Green and Associates specializes in education and policy consulting on transgender and transsexual issues. For years he was president of Female to Male International. *www.jamisongreencom, www.ftmi.org.*

MAKE-UP

Anyone with access to a computer can find assistance from licensed professionals as well as talented amateurs in every field and subject. Especially helpful are videos presented on YouTube, Vimeo and other sites. Make-up videos, both male to female and female to male, are hugely popular. Perhaps you've even made one yourself. I welcome you to share your favorite instructional videos with me by sending a link to *missvera@missvera.com.*

The Beauty Department, a site with excellent photo tutorials for different areas of make-up application. Their tutorial on highlight and contour makes that important process so clear and understandable the tutorial is helpful whether you want to enhance your current gender, or cross gender. *www.thebeautydepartment.com.*

Books offer the advantage of staying open on a page, so you can take your time in learning without having to stop, back up and hit replay.

Kevyn AuCoin, *Making Faces.* AuCoin is now a make-up saint but his books live on as make-up bibles.

Bobbi Brown. *Bobbi Brown Make Up Manual,* reviewed by laura m2F, who says she loved it.

Dita von Teese. *Your Beauty Mark: The Ultimate Guide to Eccentric Glamour.* Dita, strip artiste and model, was like me mentored by Ms. Antoinette. A gossipy gorgeous book. Dita lets you into her life and shares her considerable expertise.

MONEY

Suze Orman. *www.SuzeOrman.com.*

SCORE. Need a business mentor? The SCORE Association, "Counselors to America's Small Business," is a nonprofit association comprised of 13,000+ volunteer business counselors throughout the U.S. and its territories. Many are retired executives. SCORE members are trained to serve as counselors, advisors and mentors to aspiring entrepreneurs and business owners. These services are offered at no fee, as a community service. 320 chapters, plus online help. *www.score.org.*

Debtors Anonymous and Business Debtors Anonymous.
Whether you are a college graduate with a mountain of student loan debt, a struggling small business owner, or simply a person who just can't seem to earn more than you spend, twelve-step programs like DA, Business Debtors Anonymous (BDA) or Under Earners Anonymous can help, and meetings are free. Lots of meetings all over and telephone meetings too. *www.debtorsanonymous.org, www.underearnersanonymous.org*

SEXUALITY

Betty Dodson. As a solo artist Betty Dodson has had a profound influence on our sexuality, through her visual art, books such as *Liberating Masturbation,* and bodysex workshops. Ten years ago Betty teamed up with dedicated and internet-savvy Carlin Ross; together they have created a blog, advice column and e-zine of immense value in the present and for future generations. *www.dodsonandross.com.*

Center For Sex and Culture. 1349 Mission Street, San Francisco. Founded by author Dr. Carol Queen and Dr. Robert Lawrence. Resource center, archive, hotbed of a wide variety of exciting, educational and erotic events. *www.sexandculture.org.*

Urban Tantra, by Barbara Carrellas. Barbara puts it all together: breath, energy, gender fluidity, tantra, polyamory, kink. She sees the big picture. Barbara goes around the world teaching others, including other sex educators. *www.barbaracarrellas.com.*

The Ultimate Guide to Kink, by Tristin Taormino. It took a special person to bring anal sex into public discussion and Tristan did it with wit, intelligence, and courage. She's a whip-smart champion of sexual freedom and understanding.

Jackie A. Castro. Her two books *Fetish and Him,* which she wrote for partners, and *Fetish and You* validate sexual uniqueness. She is a psychotherapist in private practice. *www.therapywithcare.com.*

Museum of Sex. 233 Fifth Avenue, NYC. Covers art, porn, human practices. The top floor that describes variety in the animal world is truly mind-expanding. *www.museumofsex.com.*

SexEcology. "Earth as lover not mother," say the ecosexuals Annie Sprinkle and Elizabeth Stephens. Find out more on their website, which includes videos of their marriages to the Earth. Screen "Good-Bye Gauley Mountain: An Ecosexual Love Story." *www.sexecology.org.*

International Professional Surrogates Association. *www.surrogate-therapy.org.* The movie *The Sessions,* starring Helen Hunt, shone light on the valuable contributions of sex surrogates with a compassionate hands-on approach.

Tamar and Ray Reilly, doctors of human sexuality, practice mainly in the Los Angeles area. They have my highest recommendations. www.thesexsurrogate.com

Gloria G. Brame, Ph.D. Therapist, sexologist and author. The landmark book *Different Loving* is just one of her many books. Just completed is *A Different Loving, Too.* Her blogs are full of great information and humor. *www.gloriabrame.com.*

American Association of Sex Educators, Counselors and Therapists. Sexologist and Therapists. Not every therapist is sex-positive. This website has a helpful directory. *www.aasect.org.*

MONOGAMY AND POLYAMORY

Designer Relationships. By Mark A. Michaels and Patricia Johnson. (Cleis Press). One of many books from this couple. *www.tantrapm.com.*

SEXUALITY BOUTIQUES

Thanks to dedicated sex educators and entrepreneurs, couple-friendly sexuality boutiques exist in most major cities across this country and internationally. Many of the shops have guest speakers and run classes, and most have online stores. Here are just a few. Write to me to tell me about shops near you.

www.Babeland.com. See "Gender Expression" category.

www.goodvibes.com

www.HustlerHollywood.com

www.thepleasurechest.com

www.sexploratorium.net, in Philadelphia.

The Center For Sex and Health. Pawtucket, Rhode Island. Besides their own location, you can put "sexuality shops" in their search engine and find other shops in the U.S. and Canada. *www.thecsph.org.*

SHOPPING FOR WARDROBE

Shopping for clothes has never been easier. Most stores, particularly department stores are aware a segment of their customers want to try on cross gender options and they have trained their staffs to accommodate the needs of all customers.

Don't be afraid to ask for the try-on facility you need.

Whether you are shopping online or in a store, the first step is to know your measurements. Measure your body so that you can compare your measurements with those of the garment. Most online stores provide a size chart. Be sure to check the size chart for that particular item because sizes vary depending on the manufacturer. Some manufacturers give a more generous cut. A size 12 dress or 42 jacket might fit perfectly from one company but you might be swimming in the same size from a different manufacturer.

Shopping in a store and actually trying on the garment is best. However, that is not always convenient. Take your measurements with you, plus a measuring tape. With your tape, you will measure the garment and compare with your own numbers.

How to measure:

Shoulder: From shoulder tip to shoulder tip.

Sleeve: From underarm to wrist/end of cuff.

Hip: Measure the point of your hips that meets the top of your legs. This is usually about 9 inches below your waist.

Inside Leg (inseam of garment): The distance from your crotch to your ankle.

Length: Length of garment. Lengths are taken from the highest point of the back of the garment, the shoulder or neckline, to the hem. How does the length of the garment compare with your height?

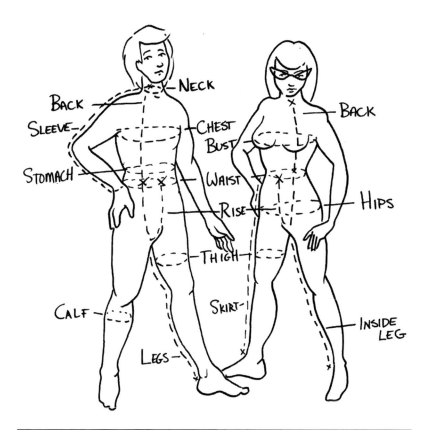

Will you need to hem the garment? Most garments don't have a lot of extra material in the hem, so if that dress or those trousers seem to short, best to not buy.

Bust: Measure around the fullest part of your bust. If you are going male to female, be sure to measure with breast forms in place.

Waist: The slimmest part of your natural waistline – above your navel and below your rib cage. Elastic in the waistband is helpful particularly if you are going male to female and need a larger waist, but don't want the hips in the garment to be too large.

Rise: This is the distance from the top of the waistband to the crotch. This corresponds to your belly area. It's an important measurement when you are purchasing jeans or other trousers. No one of any gender wants to have a crotch that digs in.

Classic Curves. There are many places online where you can shop to enhance your figure. One of our favorites sites is by Espy Lopez at *www.clcrv.com*.

ILLUSTRATION & PHOTO ACKNOWLEDGMENTS

Illustrator: Kate Devereux Smith. Kate, a self-taught artist, was mentored by Stuart Cottingham. Her interest these days is in mastering the art of tattoo. Bodies are her canvas.

Additional Illustration: Miss Vera's Academy Crest designed by Viqui Sue Maggio, my very first "Deputy Headmistress" and "Dean of Etiquette." *www.maggiographics.com*.

Photographers:

Annie Sprinkle. "Trash" and "Shelly, Queen of Clubs" are part of Annie Sprinkle's Post Porn Modernist Playing Cards. "The Seven Men in Katharine (Gates)" is a collaboration. Katharine wrote the text, Annie took the photos, both styled the looks. Annie Sprinkle has been actively involved in the art of transformation personally and professionally in many ways throughout her life. *www.anniesprinkle.org*.

Katharine Gates. This publisher and designer has been making the world safe for deviant art. *www.gatesofheck.com*.

Rene "IATBA" Moncada designed the Post Porn Modernist Manifesto in 1989. I wrote the manifesto to commemorate the premiere of Annie's Sprinkle's show *Post Porn Modernist*. Signed by me, Rene, Annie, Candida Royalle, Frank Moore, Betty Dodson, Tuppy Owens, Michele Capozzi and others. *www.reneiamthebestartist.com*

Abe Frajndlich. From a feature on Miss Vera's Finishing School in *Elle U.K.* *www.abefoto.com*.

Philippe Vogelenzang. Thanks to the persistence of dear Philippe, Miss Vera students and deans became supermodels for a feature about our school in *Candy,* "the first transversal style magazine," published with love by visionary Luis Venegas. *www.phillippevogelenzang.com, www.candy.byluisvenegas.com*.

Jennifer James Byrnes. (R.I.P.) For Jennifer James's 40th birthday, I devised a photo shoot that took her from baby to bride and beyond. Photos by Annie Sprinkle. When I created Miss Vera's Finishing School, Jennifer was our number one cheerleader. Brava and Bravo, sweet sissy.

Mariette Pathy Allen. I have called photographer Mariette "the Margaret Mead of trans." Her art and documentation helped form the movement. She is also the keeper of the Vicky West archive. Vicky was the illustrator of Lee Brewster's very influential magazine, *DRAG*. *www.mariettepathyallen.com*.

Master Zorro. Husband to Ms. Antoinette. The couple created a kinky conglomerate that consisted of magazines, *Reflections* and *Kinky Contacts*, as well as videos, fashions, and galas that helped to educate and liberate many.

Ying Ang. Ying took Miss Vera's Finishing School on as a project while a student at the renowned International Center for Photography. It was a win-win situation. We got wonderful photos of our academy life and Ying became class valedictorian. We're so proud of her as she continues her art. *www.yingangphoto.com.*

Judy Schiller. Photographer Judy inspired our student Bianca with great directions. It's not surprising that after rich career in photography capturing jazz greats, plus Nelson Mandela and other leaders and notables, Judy is now adding documentary filmmaker to her credits. *www.fotoqueen.com*

Julia Bingham. Miss Julia is dean of high heels at Miss Vera's Finishing School. She studied dance and earned a degree in theater arts while a student in Moscow. Julia understands the importance of photography in the creation of our students' cross gender identities.

Barbara Nitke. In her magnificent memoir *American Ecstasy,* Barbara Nitke documents her years as a porn movie set photographer. Her other major work is with BDSM couples. She is trusted in the most intimate moments. She photographed Michelle, one of our earliest students, and others. *www.barbaranitke.com.*

Sophia Wallace. Sophia Wallace is a conceptual artist and photographer, best known for her Cliteracy project. She champions women's rights to freedom of sexuality. She's also my cousin, of whom I'm very proud. I called in Sophia to photograph students in various fashions and poses, including a reach for Marsha's own inner clitoris. *www.sophiawallace.com.*

Daphne Chan. Canadian artist Daphne won a grant for *Transparency: The Gender Identity Project,* but she fell in love with New York and has remained. *www.DaphneChan.com.*

Dr. Kit Rachlin took the photo of Johnny Science and also found a home for Johnny's archives at Fales Library, NYU. Photos courtesy Dr. Kit Rachlin and Chris Straayer, Assoc. Prof. NYU. *www.katherinerachlin.com.*

ABOUT THE AUTHOR ƚUOꓭA ꓤOHƚUA ƎHƚ

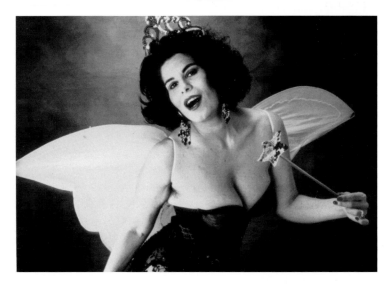

Miss Vera as Fairy Godmother. Photo by Eric Kroll.

DR. VERONICA VERA MADE HISTORY when she opened Miss Vera's Finishing School for Boys Who Want to Be Girls in New York City in 1992. The world's first crossdressing academy has become internationally famous since that day, offering a much-needed service to the vast transgender community. Miss Vera, a groundbreaking authority in the area of gender issues and sexuality in general, has authored three books on the subject, appeared on more than fifty television shows, and been the focus of countless radio interviews, magazine, newspaper, and online articles.

Today, Miss Vera has expanded her academy to include women, couples and non-binary individuals. She believes that since life is art, it's best lived with tolerance, creativity and flair.

CONNECT WITH MISS VERA

Individuals, couples and groups who wish to be guided by me and Miss Vera's Finishing School through the process of discovering a cross gender self are invited to visit *www.missvera.com,* where you will find information in how to enroll for in-person classes or phone/internet guidance. You will also find the link to our channel on youtube and my blog posts.

To book Dr. Veronica Vera for a presentation at your college or social group, please contact *missvera@missvera.com.*

To subscribe to Miss Vera's newsletter, please email *missvera@ missvera.com.*

Veronica Vera on twitter: *@MissVera212.*

I would so love to meet each of you personally to plan a curriculum devoted to your needs, and to guide you through this exciting process of transformation and integration. But I know that is not always possible. It makes me happy to be able to reach you through this book. My two previous books are *Miss Vera's Finishing School for Boys Who Want to Be Girls* (Main Street Books, 1997) and *Miss Vera's Cross Dress For Success* (Broadway Books 2002), also available as an e-book.

BDSM/KINK

The Artisan's Book of Fetishcraft: Patterns and Instructions for Creating Professional Fetishwear, Restraints & Equipment
John Huxley $27.95

At Her Feet: Powering Your Femdom Relationship
TammyJo Eckhart and Fox $14.95

Conquer Me: girl-to-girl wisdom about fulfilling your submissive desires
Kacie Cunningham $13.95

Family Jewels: A Guide to Male Genital Play and Torment
Hardy Haberman $12.95

Flogging
Joseph Bean $11.95

The Human Pony: A Guide for Owners, Trainers and Admirers
Rebecca Wilcox $27.95

Intimate Invasions: The Ins and Outs of Erotic Enema Play
M.R. Strict $13.95

The Mistress Manual: a good girl's guide to female dominance
Mistress Lorelei Powers $16.95

The (New and Improved) Loving Dominant
John Warren $16.95

The New Bottoming Book
The New Topping Book
Dossie Easton & Janet W. Hardy $14.95 ea.

Playing Well With Others: Your Field Guide to Discovering, Exploring and Navigating the Kink, Leather and BDSM Communities
Lee Harrington & Mollena Williams $19.95

Play Piercing
Deborah Addington $13.95

Radical Ecstasy: SM Journeys to Transcendence
Dossie Easton & Janet W. Hardy $16.95

The Seductive Art of Japanese Bondage
Midori, photographs by Craig Morey $27.95

The Sexually Dominant Woman: A Workbook for Nervous Beginners
Lady Green $11.95

SM 101: A Realistic Introduction
Jay Wiseman $24.95

Spanking for Lovers
Janet W. Hardy $15.95

GENERAL SEXUALITY

A Hand in the Bush: The Fine Art of Vaginal Fisting
Deborah Addington $13.95

The Jealousy Workbook: Exercises and Insights for Managing Open Relationships
Kathy Labriola $19.95

Love In Abundance: A Counselor's Advice on Open Relationships
Kathy Labriola $15.95

Phone Sex: Oral Skills and Aural Thrills
Miranda Austin $15.95

Tricks... To Please a Man
Tricks... To Please a Woman
both by Jay Wiseman $13.95 ea.

When Someone You Love Is Kinky
Dossie Easton & Catherine A. Liszt $15.95

TOYBAG GUIDES:
A Workshop In A Book   **$9.95 each**

Age Play, by Lee "Bridgett" Harrington

Basic Rope Bondage, by Jay Wiseman

Chastity Play, by Miss Simone

Clips and Clamps, by Jack Rinella

Dungeon Emergencies & Supplies, by Jay Wiseman

Hot Wax and Temperature Play, by Spectrum

Playing With Taboo, by Mollena Williams

Greenery Press books are available from your favorite on-line or brick-and-mortar bookstore or erotic boutique. These and other Greenery Press books are also available in ebook format from all major ebook retailers.

NOTES

NOTES